UP FROM DOWN UNDER

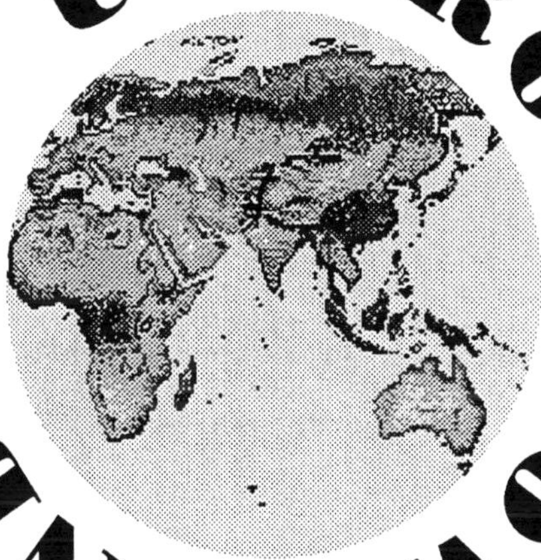

Published by Rosslyn McLeod,

P.O. Box 277, Canterbury,

Victoria , Australia 3126

First printing (Australia)	July 1994
Second printing (Australia)	October 1994
Second edition (Great Britain)	January 1995
Third edition (Australia)	May 1995

Printed by Alphagraphics , Melbourne.

ISBN 0 646 195689

UP FROM DOWN UNDER

THE AUSTRALIAN ORIGINS OF
FREDERICK MATTHIAS ALEXANDER
and
THE ALEXANDER TECHNIQUE

by

ROSSLYN McLEOD

CONTENTS

ILLUSTRATIONS

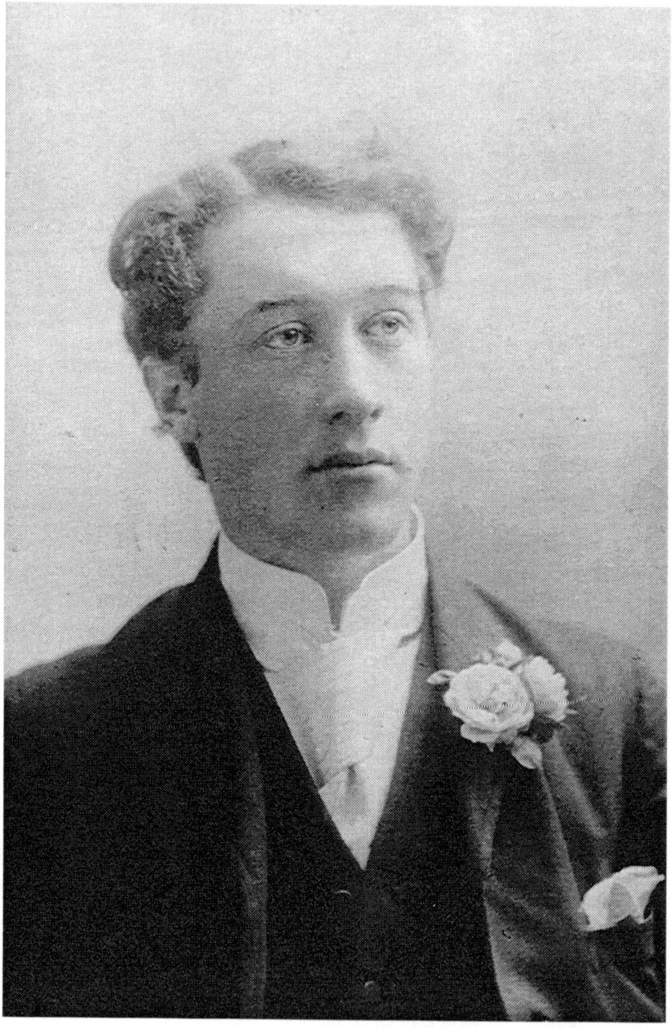

F. M. Alexander. A studio portrait, Hobart, 1894 (Courtesy of Mary Scott)

FOREWORD

Rosslyn McLeod's researches into the life of F.M.Alexander, known to Alexander teachers as 'FM', have occupied her for many years, in the intervals of her busy life as a musician and Alexander teacher. Her quest brought her some years ago to Trinity College in the University of Melbourne in order to pursue details of F.M.Alexander's correspondence with my predecessor, the first Warden of Trinity, Dr.Alexander Leeper. As the present book shows, Dr.Leeper greatly valued Alexander's philosophy and approach, and recommended that his methods should be taught in all Victorian schools rather than a rival school of 'physical culture', which was concerned more with developing muscles than with the living and breathing whole person. We are left wondering how differently things might have turned out if only Dr.Leeper's Report had been adopted by the government of the day.

There are now thousands of teachers and pupils in many countries who are grateful for the natural methods, based on acute observation, discovered and systematised by F.M.Alexander. They will be fascinated by Rosslyn McLeod's lively account of the historical, social, and cultural context in which their founder grew up, worked, and made his discoveries. Largely, no doubt because of films, television serials, and sporting successes, Australia has recently become a country of world-wide interest. F.M.Alexander may be one of Australia's less well known heroes - indeed, much of his teaching life was spent in London - but there can be no doubt about the importance of his Australian origins and upbringing to his success and therefore to his steadily growing influence.

This book portrays both the man and the country of his birth and his professional development. We see him as an elocutionist and actor who developed his famous 'technique' in response to his own problems with a faltering voice. In time, he concentrated on teaching rather than performing, and so influenced for good far more people than he would ever have delighted from the stage or platform. Even readers who know a good deal of Australian history will be both instructed and delighted by Rosslyn's vivid pictures of life in remote northern Tasmania, in Victoria during the gold rushes, 'Marvellous Melbourne' in the 1880's, and later in Hobart, New Zealand, and Sydney, where Alexander attracted large and enthusiastic audiences for his dramatic recitations, while offering lessons in breathing and voice production.

We find that he had acquired his skill as a teacher by being appointed a 'monitor' at the age of only fourteen to assist the local schoolmaster in Wynyard. Later he became an accountant at the Mt.Bischoff tin mine, which had only recently been connected to the port at Burnie by telegraph and railway. He might have remained permanently in remote obscurity with his account books, except for the happy discovery that he could entertain the other workers by giving recitations. He was attracted to Melbourne, which thanks to all that gold could buy, had become a glittering cultural capital where his talents could flourish.

This wonderful story awaits discovery in the following pages. My predecessor, Dr.Leeper, was privileged to meet F.M.Alexander and to receive lessons from him. I am privileged to have read in manuscript, and to be invited to introduce, this account by an Alexander teacher from a later generation, who has deep respect for the work of F.M.Alexander.

Evan L. Burge
Fifth Warden of Trinity College,
The University of Melbourne, Australia.

4 July 1994

PREFACE TO THE THIRD EDITION

Since the first publication of this book in July 1994 there has been an increase in research relating to Frederick Matthias Alexander, his life and work. I have been encouraged by the response to my original publication and as a result of further work I now print this Third Edition, which will be my final major contribution in this sphere. For this printing I wish to give special thanks to Mr Jean Fischer of England for his assistance, and for his kind permission to quote complete and partial extracts from certain articles and pamphlets by F M Alexander. Research takes time, but can bring its own rewards. Looking at the newspapers and magazines in Australia and New Zealand of one hundred years ago has given me clearer insight into that era. I hope the material in this book will convey to readers something of the atmosphere of that bygone age in which Frederick Matthias Alexander began his journey of personal experiment and discovery.

Rosslyn McLeod
May 1995

INTRODUCTION

At the time of writing (July, 1994) there is no biography of F.M.Alexander, although there are more than twenty books on the work that Alexander developed, known as the Alexander Technique. We are products of our time. Each life is shaped by three main influences: heredity, our individual ancestral stock; environment, where we grow up, people we are in contact with; and thirdly, use, the way in which we choose to carry out the detail of our lives, the mental, emotional and physical minutiae that shape what we become. It is the third influence, USE, and how we deal with it, that came to occupy F.M.Alexander for much of his life.

Frederick Matthias Alexander came from a family with a rich history of trial, tribulation and success. He grew up in Tasmania, an island renowned for its rugged beauty and scenic grandeur, with a short and turbulent history of white settlement. Enterprise and self-reliance were the attributes which enabled people to improve their lot.

Very few people reach their full potential as performers, whether it be in the artistic field, sport or some other endeavour. The reasons will vary; lack of commitment, not having the lucky breaks despite the hours of study or training. How students think about what they are doing, how they interpret the advice of teachers; the teacher's own background and knowledge, and the way they explain things; all this goes into the making of a performer. When performance is marred, for whatever reason, many give up, and decide to try something else. Alexander was a stayer; he had voice problems, and he didn't want to give up. His uniqueness is in the way he solved his own problems and then translated this experience into teaching others the fundamentals of the Use of the Self, which enable each individual to realise more of his or her potential in a given activity.

Times change. We can only view past lives through understanding something of their environment. We can never totally experience a past era. Looking back is always tinged, to a greater or lesser degree, with knowledge of the present. Since the 1988 Bicentenary in Australia there has been much more awareness of the value of old documents; perhaps in the future material will be brought forward that may throw more light on the early days of F.M.Alexander's teaching in Australia. What follows is an outline of his origins, his life here and the beginnings of his teaching; the telling of a fuller story is for some future historian.

EARLY AUSTRALIA

Terra Australis Incognita, the Unknown South Land

For centuries, Terra Australis Incognita - the Unknown South Land, had been one of the great mysteries for sailors and traders who ventured from Europe to far-flung parts of the world. The Portuguese, Spanish and Dutch were the first to explore the general area, followed in the eighteenth century by the French and British. Small sections of the Australian coastline had become known but it was Captain James Cook, commissioned by the British Government to explore in the region, who charted much of the east coast of Australia and claimed it as a British possession in 1770 under *'the name of New South Wales'*.

There were several main reasons for the British establishing such an outpost so far from the mother country. After the American War of Independence (1776) Britain could no longer send her prison surplus to America. Rather than build more gaols in England the authorities looked for other areas to transport their convicts. Captain Cook and other members of his party had reported favourably on the condition of the New South Wales land that they had seen in 1770. The British Government concluded that survival of convicts in this new settlement would be possible.

Other reasons for Britain establishing a colony on the east coast of Australia were to provide the home country with:

1. a maritime base as a staging post for their shipping routes in the Pacific - including ship repair and maintenance.
2. new sources of timber and flax. These were basic materials for ships and sea-power was critical for a nation to maintain supremacy. Australia seemed a good, possible provider of these materials.
3. protection and safety for the increase of its trade in the general region.

The First Fleet

In 1788, the British Government sent the First Fleet under the command of Captain Arthur Philip to New South Wales. It was a very expensive exercise. Just over one thousand people were in that first contingent, about three quarters of them convicts, the rest mainly officers and men to guard the felons, and a few skilled tradesmen.

In order to become self-sufficient as quickly as possible the most urgent task was to start growing crops. Supplementary supplies from Britain would take eight months to a year to reach the colony, given the hazardous nature of long sea voyages, and arrivals would be unreliable. As well as the planting of crops, adequate water supplies had to be found, some form of housing, however primitive, erected, and suitable land prepared on which to run the European animals brought with the First Fleet.

The first few years of the colony's life were often desperate times - severe rationing had to be introduced, thieving and drunkenness were rife and the newcomers were unaccustomed to the harshness of the weather. The hardships of the early settlers were gradually overcome, the town of Sydney grew and the tents and flimsy huts were replaced by houses of brick or stone. With exploration of the surrounding country, fertile land was found which allowed for more intensive farming, though this was still difficult because of the shortage of farm implements.

As more people came from Britain to the colony there was an increase in the number of free settlers. They came as a result of pleas to the British Government by the early Governors of New South Wales, who saw that sustained development of the new settlement as a viable community needed people with various skills (particularly agricultural) who were willing to work hard. Many of the convicts sent out proved unwilling labourers and chose to continue a life of crime, while others did change, secured tickets-of-leave, took up farming or other occupations and became respected citizens.

As well as the exploration of land around Sydney, there grew a curiosity about the southern part of Australia. Back in 1642 the Dutchman, Abel Tasman, had discovered part of a land mass which he called Van Diemen's Land, (now Tasmania). Little further exploration was made in this area until in 1798 Bass and Flinders left Sydney to investigate the region in detail. In an epic voyage they circumnavigated Van Diemen's Land. On their return to Sydney, Bass and Flinders gave reports of the extensive whale and seal colonies they had seen in what became known as Bass Strait. This often rough, treacherous stretch of water between southern Australia and northern Tasmania has proved to be the graveyard for many ships.

In 1801 Flinders published an account of this voyage, titled,

" Observations on the coasts of

VAN DIEMEN'S LAND,

on

BASS'S STRAIT and its ISLANDS

and on part of the coast of

NEW SOUTH WALES

intended to accompany the

CHARTS OF THE LATE DISCOVERIES

in those countries

By Matthew Flinders

Second Lieutenant of His Majesty's Ship Reliance

LONDON

Printed by John Nichols

Earl's Court, Little Newport Street, Soho
1801

On passing the Table Cape area of North West Tasmania (where the Alexanders were to settle in the 1840's) Flinders wrote:

"The bight between Circular Head and the next projection eastward, is almost entirely a sandy beach; and there are also sandy beaches half way from the rocky projection towards Table Cape; but the shore then becomes rocky and steep. Both Circular Head and Table Cape, and also the rocky cape between them, make like islands when first seen from the eastward. The Table Cape preserves its flat appearance in every direction from the sea. Its cliffs are steep; and it is high enough to be seen at the distance of twelve leagues."

News of the rich sea life in Bass Strait encouraged whalers and sealers to move into the area. They used some coastal parts of Van Diemen's Land as temporary shore bases and the industry became a valuable one for New South Wales. In 1803 a small permanent settlement, called Hobart Town was begun on the shore of the Derwent River in the southern part of the island. This was established partly because Britain was wary of the French surveying of the coastline. In 1806 a second settlement was established by the British in northern Van Diemen's Land at what is now Launceston. Both settlements were organised separately and no attempt was made for some years to explore the country between the two; communication was by sea and both were controlled from Sydney.

By 1809 the population of New South Wales, (ie., the whole known mainland of Australia) was 10,000, with another 1,300 people in the two settlements in Van Diemen's Land. The early struggles and hardships of New South Wales now gave way to more sustained development. Life was still difficult but for those willing to work there were increasing opportunities for advancement. Explorers ventured further into the hinterland, opening up vast tracts for sheep, cattle and wheat. Roads were built, trade flourished, the business and commercial district of Sydney developed. Fine buildings were erected. Though convicts continued to form a large part of the population for some time, there was an increasing number of native-born people known as Currency lads and lassies, who were respected as being mostly hard-working and self-reliant.

Van Diemen's Land

In 1820 Van Diemen's Land had 3,000 convicts, almost half of the total population. To help ease the shortage of labour on the island, an increasing number of convicts was sent from Britain, though the convict percentage in relation to the island's total population declined. In 1825 Van Diemen's Land became a colony separate from New South Wales, with a Lieutenant-Governor responsible to the Colonial Office in London. Hobart, growing in importance, became the colony's capital. For some years it was the greatest whaling port in the South Pacific, and a vital shipbuilding industry was developed, which by the 1840's was larger than that of the other five mainland Australian colonies put together.

The Aborigines

The first Australians, the Aborigines, had been living on this Continent for many thousands of years. Their way of life was tribal, no individual owned any land, everything was shared. The tribes were highly organised and had their own languages and customs; their basic needs of food were supplied by hunting and food-gathering - not by cultivation of permanent crops; they were nomads, each group moving within certain territorial boundaries so there was no need of permanent shelter.

The first documented evidence of contact between white people and the Australian Aborigines was by seafarers exploring parts of the Australian coastline in the early seventeenth century. In 1770 Captain James Cook noted the contacts he had made with the Aborigines whilst exploring the east coast of Australia.

When the First Fleet came from Britain in 1788 to form the colony of New South Wales there was early contact between whites and blacks. How these contacts have subsequently developed for over two hundred years has been the subject of much debate and documentation. The early white settlers chose the most fertile land on which to farm their crops and animals. The Aborigines' water supplies were polluted and their food supplies destroyed.

With the passing of time, as the white settlers extended their land holdings, the Aborigines were forced to eke out their existence in the most inhospitable parts of the country. The pastoralists and later the miners used the land in ways which Aborigines had never envisaged. Inevitably, there was conflict, though some attempts were made by certain individual white people to try living harmoniously with the Aborigines and to understand their culture. In any armed struggles the whites, with their superior weapons, were the ultimate victors. It was not only the fighting that led to so many Aboriginal deaths and a swift decline in the Australian Aboriginal population. The living conditions for the Aborigines deteriorated. Their contact with white people led to infection, from various white man's diseases to which they had no immunity; to over-use of alcohol and tobacco, and adoption of the worst features of the white man's diet.

In the 1800's numerous attempts to put the Aborigines into special reservations, run either by government or various Christian missions, led to further disintegration of tribal groups. The question of Aboriginal rights and the relationship of Aborigines to white society in Australia has been and is still the subject of debate. The issues are many and complex. In mainland Australia, Aborigines, both full-blood and half-caste, have survived. Time, Government legislation and the changing attitudes of whites, have seen some improvement for the Aboriginal population.

In Tasmania the Aboriginal history is a dismal and sombre one. In less than one hundred years after white settlement (begun in 1803) the Aboriginal population, which initially was approximately 4,000, became extinct. The various Aboriginal tribes suffered defeat in battles with the whites over land settlement and use; or contracted white man's diseases. In the 1830's the last two hundred full-blood Aborigines in Van Diemen's Land were moved to Flinders Island in the eastern part of Bass Strait. The last survivors died in 1876.

The attitude of white people towards the Aborigines depended then, as it does now, upon the individual's background and upbringing. Some were sympathetic to the Aborigines, others not. Some saw the Aborigines' way of life as that of the 'noble savage' existing without the complications and trappings of white civilization; they had no farming, no domestic animals, no planting of crops, they could just be at one with Nature. Others saw the blacks as mean, despicable creatures, little better than mere animals.

Van Diemen's Land (Tasmania) in 1831

The population of Hobart was about 6,000. By now much of the interior of Van Diemen's Land had been explored and the good land opened up for farming. Farms were basically self-supporting and run by free settlers or ex-convicts who had been pardoned. Few of the convict population (numbering about 10,000) were held in confinement. They were put to work felling timber, clearing land and building roads. Apart from government projects, many were assigned to work for free settlers and officials.

There were codes of regulations regarding the treatment of convicts, the interpretation of which was variable, depending on whether the master was a good man or a hard one. Flogging was the usual punishment for misbehaviour. Sometimes, in desperation, convicts tried to escape. If they succeeded there was then the problem of how to survive in the harsh and inhospitable bush. Some became bushrangers, preying on travellers and those in isolated places, but usually not for long as capture was inevitable.

For most people in Van Diemen's Land in the 1830's life was about obtaining the necessities, food, adequate clothing and shelter, and animals, particularly bullocks and horses for transport. There were some pleasures in life, and moments of relaxation, but overall life was rough and tough.

It was into this environment that Matthias Alexander, convict, and grandfather of F. M. Alexander, arrived in Hobart Town. It was May 29th, 1831.

ENGLAND - THE ALEXANDER BROTHERS

The Old World and the New

Transportation had become the accepted way for Britain to rid her shores of those in society who transgressed, for one reason or another. The justification for the convict system and the deplorable conditions under which it was carried out became the subject of increasing debate, both in Britain and Australia. One social group in Britain which suffered especially from difficult living conditions was the farm labourers. Their plight grew ever more desperate in the late 1820's and in 1830 led to a series of riots in many counties which became known as the 'Swing Riots'.

The agricultural system in Britain was comprised of three sections: a few owners of large tracts of land; a middle group of farmers and tenant-farmers; and the largest and most economically disadvantaged group, the farm labourers who worked for wages on a yearly or casual weekly/daily basis. Unrest amongst this last group was fuelled by appallingly low wages, high rents, uncertain employment prospects and a minimal system of social security. A combination of social injustice, harsh climatic conditions, the introduction of threshing machines which replaced mens' labour, a change of government in Britain, and political disquiet in France and Belgium, all pointed towards change. The villages became places of rumour and expectation.

When discontent turned to active protest, isolated actions ignited similar protests that swept through county after county. The type and severity of action taken by the farm labourers varied considerably. There was arson and threatening letters - usually with the signature 'Mr. Swing', or'Captain Swing', or 'Swing', which led to the riots of 1830 becoming known as the 'Captain Swing riots'. There was display of intimidating handbills and posters, meetings re demands for higher wages, assaults on overseers, parsons and landlords, and destruction of different types of machinery, particularly the threshing machines. The majority of people involved in the protests were the farm labourers but others too gave active support, including various skilled craftsmen.

The county of Wiltshire suffered especially from social injustice. Wages were very low. The destruction of the threshing machines became a particular target for agitators. When those guilty of this crime or other disturbances were caught, tried and found guilty of 'machine-breaking', many were sentenced to transportation to the Colonies of Australia. Most (330 men) were sent to Van Diemen's Land and a smaller number to New South Wales. Matthias Alexander, the grandfather of F.M.Alexander, was one of those sent to Van Diemen's Land on the ship 'Eliza'. All two hundred and twenty-four convicts on board arrived safely in Hobart on May 29th 1831. This was an unusual occurrence. Because of appalling conditions deaths on the way out were all too common. Van Diemen's Land at this time had a total population of 25,000, forty per cent of whom were convicts.

Living conditions aboard the convict ships were basic. Food was just adequate, the below deck sleeping berths allowed each man eighteen inches of space, nearly always there was poor ventilation. Prisoners were on deck for daily exercise if weather permitted, handcuffed together and secured by leg irons. If the weather was inclement prisoners had to stay below deck in the foul atmosphere. This could be for days on end. The 'Eliza' took one hundred and twelve days to make the journey from Portsmouth to Hobart.

On arrival in Hobart the convicts were checked, taken ashore and assigned for service with either government or private employers, such as landowners or farmers. Generally the 'machine-breakers' were regarded as being of better moral character than the normal run of convicts. A campaign to secure an amnesty for the 'machine-breakers' built up in Britain in the early 1830's, and from 1835 to 1837 successive issues of free pardons were made to these people.

Transportation of convicts from Britain to Australia had begun in 1788. In her earlier history Australia had relied heavily on convict labour but as the number of free settlers and native-born people increased so opposition grew to this form of cheap labour. As well, in both Britain and Australia there was increasing pressure to abandon this form of treatment for wrongdoers on humanitarian grounds .Transportation of convicts to New South Wales ceased in 1840, other colonies gradually followed suit, until finally in 1868 Western Australia was the last colony to cease transportation. This was eighty years after the first convicts had arrived in New South Wales in 1788.

The Alexanders - a new start

Matthias Alexander was born in 1810 in Wiltshire, Britain, the third child of Edward and Jane Alexander. When Matthias, aged twenty, was sentenced to Van Diemen's Land for seven years for being involved in the 'Swing riots', his older brother Joseph was similarly sentenced. The two arrived in Hobart in 1831. Later, a younger brother, John, was convicted for allegedly stealing some pigs and also received a seven year transportation sentence. This was supposedly done so he could be with his brothers.

Joseph and Matthias Alexander were pardoned in 1836. After working for a few years on an Estate in the north of the Colony they moved to the North West coast and settled in the Table Cape/Wynyard area. Still today there are descendents of the original Alexander families living in the region. The younger brother John was given a certificate of freedom in 1846. News of the gold strikes in California inspired him to seek his fortune there, then when gold was found at Ballarat in Victoria, John Alexander returned to Australia. He went to the Ballarat diggings, where he succeeded in making enough money to return to the North West of Tasmania. He became at one stage the biggest landowner at Table Cape.

GOLD GOLD

The cry of GOLD was to echo around much of the Australian continent from 1850 to 1900. It held the promise of quick financial gain, of untold wealth. Some of the gold finds drew hundreds of people, other areas attracted thousands; as more and more new sites were discovered, gold fever affected people from all walks of life.

It was known for a long time that small amounts of gold had been found in various parts of Australia, but no one made a fuss about it. In the late 1840's a great number of people, including many Australians, went to California to make their fortune when gold was discovered there. A few of the Australians who went over realised that the countryside in California where gold was discovered had similar characteristics to some of the terrain back home. Returning home these people used their prospecting skills to make successful gold finds - first in New South Wales in early 1851, later in Victoria.

The initial strikes in New South Wales drew people from neighbouring Victoria. The Victorian authorities were fearful that the colony, which had just become independent from New South Wales in 1850, would lose most of its able-bodied men to the New South Wales gold-fields. They need not have worried. When gold was discovered in Victoria it brought such a huge influx of people that Victoria's population of 87,000 in 1851 jumped to 540,000 by 1861. The capital of the Colony, Melbourne, expanded so quickly that by 1861 it easily surpassed the population of Sydney, the capital of the mother-colony of New South Wales.

Melbourne became the setting-off point for most of the gold-seekers, who were bent on travelling inland to the diggings as fast as possible. At first people came from the other Australian colonies, but as news of the rich finds reached Europe and other parts of the world, thousands set out with high hopes of finding gold and making a new start in life. Most were from the United Kingdom, other countries included China, Germany, America and France.

Ships crowded into Port Phillip Bay, eager passengers went ashore only to find Melbourne stretched to the limits to provide even basic necessities. Accommodation that was affordable was mostly in tents in an area by the side of the Yarra River known as Canvas Town. But the stay was only temporary as people quickly sought to equip themselves for one purpose only - to find gold. Once provisions were acquired they immediately set out on foot, or if they could afford it by horse, for one of the increasing number of sites that gave promise of reward and a bright prosperous future. Many crews jumped ship to head for the diggings; men left their jobs as policemen, teachers, clerks, farm labourers, servants; all enticed by the lure of the magic word GOLD.

One of the main daily newspapers in Melbourne, The Argus, printed graphic accounts each day of the latest gold finds. The following are extracts from these reports, taken from September 20th to September 27th, 1851, when GOLD was at the beginning of its long and prosperous reign in Victoria.

Each day there was a report from the Geelong correspondent. (Geelong is 72 kilometres south-west of Melbourne and after Melbourne was the next most popular place for people to go ashore when they arrived in Victoria.)

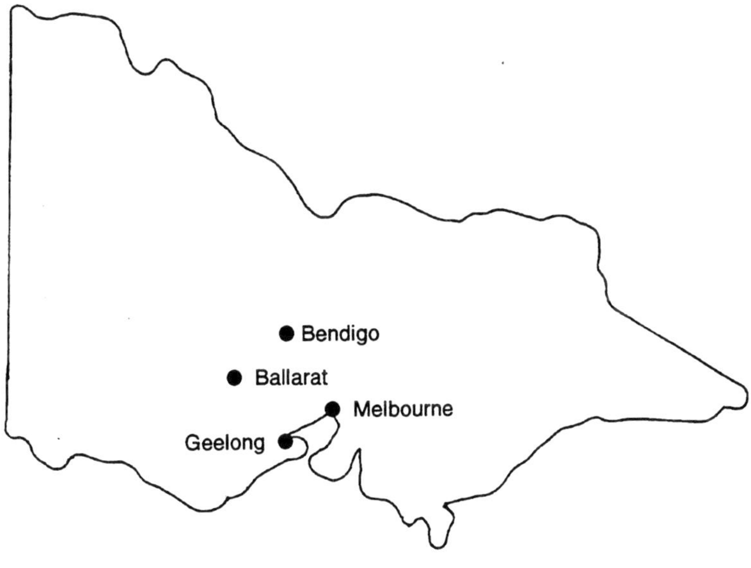

Victoria

Geelong Report, Saturday, September 20th, 1851:

"Notwithstanding the fearful inclemency of the weather - the cry is still 'they go'. The old fashioned flash expression of 'when did you come out?' has given way to the modern one of 'when are you going?' and it is so well understood, that no one ever thinks of asking to what place the question applies. If the present migration of males continues much longer, Geelong will be entirely under petticoat Government.
(Author's note; at the time women did not have the vote.) *Have you got your cradle ? says one, out of breath, as he meets another in the street; have you got your tools ? asks a second, - where did you buy your tarpaulin ? asks a third. These questions so continuously asked, coupled with the extraordinary demand for '`hay carts' and 'hosses' as 'ill go in harness, prove, that if Geelong was mad yesterday, it is still madder today. Nor is this excitement confined to the lower classes; doctors, lawyers, and master tradesmen are off to the Ballarat Diggings. The weather and the state of the roads are mere trifles apparently to these enthusiasts - these slaves of Old King Gold."*

Initially many of the diggers searched for the alluvial (surface) gold, which might require a small amount of digging. As this petered out, diggers formed themselves into groups; then companies with financial backers were registered, so that there was the finance and the skills to buy and work the equipment needed to go deeper and deeper below the earth's surface, to where the richer seams lay. The equipment used by the early diggers was simple, though often ingenuity was shown in inventing new variations of equipment to extract the gold.

For gold panning, a tin dish was all that was needed. Sand and or gravel from a creek bed (dry or flowing) was put in the pan and water added. The dish was rhythmically swirled around, the dirty water and grit gradually slopped over the lip of the dish, leaving the larger stones in the bottom, and most importantly the specks, or if you were lucky, larger pieces of gold, glittering in the dish.

A more sophisticated and faster way of washing the dirt, whether taken from the creek or the ground, was to use a 'cradle'. A cradle was made of wood and possibly iron, it could be about four feet long and it was placed on rockers, like a baby's old-fashioned cradle. Dirt was put into one end and water was thrown over it; the man rocked the cradle and kept washing the dirt until rocks and earth were washed away and the gold, being heavier, would remain in the bottom of the cradle.

Ballarat Diggings Report, Saturday, September 20th, 1851:

"The goldfield is extending hourly, and daily experiments tend to prove that its extent is all but illimitable. Two new machines for gold washing have been brought on the ground within a few days. One of them is already in operation; but it would be premature to pronounce on its efficacy before further trial. It is a cradle rocked to and fro by the action of a crank, supplying at the same time the requisite motion, and a plentiful supply of water, and saving much trouble and time in that one respect, but involving too much tin dish washing, which may, however, be modified by a few minor alterations. The second machine, which is spoken very highly of, is not yet in operation. Both have been constructed in Geelong.

"The 'Clunes Diggings' have removed to Ballarat, and Geelong has come up to Buninyong. Every available vehicle has been called into requisition, from a bullock dray to a wheel-barrow; and no small surprise was created the other day by the appearance of a man driving before him the last mentioned vehicle, containing his provisions and swag, which he had wheeled from Ashby to the Buninyong Gully in two days and a half. The man appeared quite fresh, and as indifferent to fatigue as the wheelbarrow itself. Another man brought his cradle from New Town (near Geelong) on his back, and the only complaint that he made was, that he was detained when leaving New Town, by a short gentleman in black, with a white neck-tie; he accused him of running away with his pulpit, but who apologised, after examining its construction, and 'bade the man God speed' - and on he sped, through mire and mud, bog and quagmire, until he reached the diggings, where it is hoped such perserverance may meet a fitting reward.

"As there are many intending gold diggers it may be advisable to state the requisites imperatively demanded to prosecute such business successfully. First of all, they must be made of gutta purcha, impervious to wet, and have the stomach of an ostrich to digest any aliment, or be content with none for an indefinite time; they must have an elastic constitution, adaptive to all circumstances, except comfortable ones - these may be left out of the category for the present. A gold digger must be a Jack of all-trades; he must be able to strip bark, fall a tree, and saw it, dig sods, make embankments, put up a hut, mend your clothes, draw firewood after chopping it, bake boil and roast, use a pick, and spade, delve, dig, and quarry, load, and unload, draw a sledge, and drive a barrow, cut paths, make roadways, puddle in mud, and splash ankle deep in water, with occasional slushings from head to foot, bear sleet and rain without flinching during the day, and sleep in damp blankets during the night, thankful that they are not entirely saturated - if ye can do all this, and have spirit enough to attempt it, and endurance enough to carry it on for three months, why there is gold and rheumatism in store for you. If you have a strong

constitution, it will make you hardy, but many will be spoiled in the experiment.

"Such are the scenes that I have witnessed, and endured, and call on others to prepare themselves for the like. Perhaps it would be advisable to get a coating of gutta purcha, which was recommended by a philanthropist at home to the starving peasantry of Ireland, in the supposition that waterproofing the external skin would prevent perspiration, and thus preventing the exudation of the animal juices, would supersede the necessity of supplying them which would cause a great saving of potatoes - a grand triumph of science during a famine."

Geelong Report, Monday, September 22nd, 1851:

" The gold excitement continues unabated, it is, in fact, on the increase, if that be possible; in every street drays may be seen loading for the golden district, shops are being shut up, employers are getting short-handed, the crisis is upon us; every additional arrival lends fury to the already devouring fire. There will be nobody to read the papers, and possibly nobody to print them. The tide of emigration never rolled so steadily to the colonies, as it now rolls from Geelong to Ballarat."

Geelong Report, Wednesday, September 24th, 1851:

"A new gold field is reported to have been discovered within 35 miles of Geelong; but although the locality is well known, it is considered prudent to say nothing about it at present, beyond that good gold has been found, and that it is generally believed there is plenty more of it.

"Were the secret divulged, we should have the Government vultures upon the unfortunate diggers directly; a very fine piece about two ounces, was found there last week, and a party of ten are about arranging to start this day."

Once a gold discovery was validated by the Government, an official agency was set up by the Gold Commissioner who was authorised by the Government to collect a set fee and give a licence to each miner. This allowed him to mine a given area of ground for a set length of time. Miners were required to show their licence at any time. The increasing of licence fees and the greater frequency and brutality of licence searches led to more and more diggers becoming angry and rebellious about what was happening. By 1854 rebellion had reached boiling point. A series of incidents resulted in over a thousand men gathering together and building a stockade. By the evening of Saturday December 2nd most had returned to rest in their tents. About one hundred and fifty armed diggers remained to guard the stockade. On 3rd

December it was overrun by the military in a surprise dawn attack in which about thirty men were killed. Though defeated, this stand by the miners, known as the Eureka Stockade, did lead to changes in the harsh laws in Victoria which had so inflamed the mining communities.

The Argus, Wednesday, September 24th, 1851:

"The following is the Form of License issued : -

Victoria Gold License.
21st September, 1851

No.
The Bearer,_______________, having paid to me the sum of fifteen shillings, on account of the Territorial Revenue, I hereby license him to dig, search for, and remove gold, on and from the District of Buninyong and Loddon, as I shall assign to him for that purpose, during the month of September, 1851. The quantity of ground allowed is eight feet square. the license to be produced when demanded by me, or any other person acting under the authority of the Government.

F.C.Doveton,
Commissioner.

No.
Gold License,
Name,
Date, 21st September, 1851. "

Sydney Gold Circular, Thursday, September 25th, 1851:

"It is a remarkable fact that every week brings new treasures to light in connexion with the extraordinary discovery that now so much engages the attention of our colonists - the first specimen of Australian gold was in the city of London yesterday; and when we consider the suspicion manifested in this City (Sydney) for several weeks after the secret was made known, it will not be surprising that John Bull, in our native land, should treat the first specimen exhibited to him as a strong attempt at a hoax - but when each succeeding ship conveys a much larger quantity of gold than the previous one, all his doubts will vanish, and his astonished eyes will awake to the truth that he possesses at the Antipodes a dependency of inestimable value. What will be his emotions when he hears that our very roads and bridges have been covered with this auriferous deposit, and that we have been actually sowing grain upon soil richly impregnated with the precious metal ? Marvellous as this may appear, it is no more strange than true."

Geelong Report, Thursday, September 25th, 1851:

"The full amount of the gold licenses, nay more than the full amount of them, has been exacted; and once more the representative of royalty, (I beg Her Majesty's pardon, for casting so base a slur on her fair name) has unfurled the banner of oppression, and calls on his myrmidons to rally round him, and support him in his attempt to establish a Reign of Terror.

"The full amount of half a month's license, is exacted from the pioneers of colonial prosperity, for nine days' work, including two Sabbaths. Regulations are promulgated that the license to search for gold is to be at the rate of one shilling per day: the Commissioner upsets these regulations, and on his own responsibility, raises the sum to nearly one shilling and sixpence per diem. The licenses bear date, the 21st September they terminate on the 30th of the same month, and must again be renewed; consequently, the Government have swindled the diggers out of six shillings per head....

"But, notwithstanding all that could be said against such a monstrous injustice, the exaction of a license is absolutely necessary; it is not the license, but the amount paid for it, that I object to, and especially at the present time. It may be easily imagined into what dreadful confusion the diggers would get; what fearful crimes would be committed by some of them, if left to administer their self-made laws and regulations. Judge Lynch would reign as triumphantly at Ballarat as he does in California; that now damned, doomed, black spot on the map of America, whose banner should be of blood, with the piratical emblem of skull and crossbones in the centre. A country boasting of freedom, becoming a nation of human butchers, converting their own streets and dwellings into human shambles. California has now become a bye-word among the civilised nations of the earth, - a thing to be spit upon, and so will Victoria, or any other gold-producing country that is badly governed. Let us, therefore, as willingly protect the Government in all prudent measure, as we would the diggers. In the course of time, perhaps a more favourable opportunity for exacting a Royalty might present itself, but at present such an imposition is impolitic, unjust, and disgraceful. I do not by any means approve of this Royalty being claimed by the Crown at any time, unless the colony receives the benefit of it, that is to say, unless the Royalty fee be appropriated to purposes connected with the welfare of the colony. ....

"Considerable quantities of gold continue to arrive in town. ....

"The general impression made upon those intelligent people who have lately visited the mines is, that one third of the diggers are making almost fortunes; one-third are making first-rate wages, and the other third are hard set to make a living - it is in fact here what it always was in other countries - a mere lottery, attended with great privations."

Geelong, (reprinted from the Geelong Advertiser), Friday, September 26th, 1851:

"The gold excitement is every day getting stronger and stronger. Respectable parties, it is true, have come down with woeful tidings of disappointment, and predict a melancholy reaction before many days. We have been asked to do what we can to stem the ruinous torrent, and gladly would we see the excitement moderated. But in the mean time, to stem the tide, or to cool down the feverish pulse, we think impossible. Every thing will find its level, and in a very short time facts and circumstances will prove to all the real state of things. At present the assertions on one side and another are so perfectly conflicting, that no party will believe unless they see or experience the facts of the case."

Editorial, The Argus, Melbourne, Saturday, September 27th,1851:

"The City was all alive, yesterday, with a report that an eminent firm in Melbourne, had purchased one lot of gold from the Ballarat diggings, to the amount of eleven hundred pounds. We have not heard whether this report be duly authenticated, but it was very generally believed. In connection with reports from other sources, there can now, we think, be no doubt whatever that the new diggings near Buninyong are of a very rich description, and that they will probably furnish a very large quantity of the precious metal opened up as their resources will be, by the hundreds rapidly flocking to the neighbourhood.

"We trust that the Government is fully aware of the state of things likely to arise, and is prepared to take measures equal to the emergency. Complete police control is of the first importance, to check any tendency to outrage to which a suddenly accumulated, and very heterogeneous mass is so prone. A large part of the crowd fast trending in that direction, will consist of men of very objectionable character, the seventy four Vandemonians (Ed., means Tasmanians), *kindly brought us by The Screw, probably amongst the number; and as all reports agree that every road is lined with fresh pilgrims to the Golden shrine, it is obvious that a body will soon be assembled, for which Captain Dana and a blackfellow or two will constitute a very inadequate protection. A bad spirit is more easily prevented than checked when once created; and we, therefore, trust that immediate measures will be taken for the full enforcement of order, and protection to life and property.*

"Periodical escorts ought also to be provided both to Melbourne and Geelong. It is highly inexpedient to allow of large accumulations of gold upon the ground, or to force its transmission along our lonely roads without protection. Either of these courses would be sure to lead to outrage, quarrel-

ling, robbery, and bloodshed; and as these are the means of converting our gold discoveries into a curse instead of a blessing, we hope to see them timely averted, by vigorous and intelligent action upon the part of the Government."

The above extracts from The Argus, a daily Melbourne newspaper, cover one week in 1851. Gold was to dominate the colony of Victoria for many years. Ballarat and the surrounding area, just over 100 kilometres northwest of the state capital, Melbourne, was one of the wealthiest and most famous of the Victorian gold regions. By October 1851 the Ballarat area had 5,000 diggers; in a few years this number was to double. It was here in the first part of the 1850's that John Alexander, brother of Matthias Alexander, found the gold that enabled him to return to Table Cape (Tasmania) and buy 1,500 acres of heavily timbered land. John's older brother Matthias (grandfather of F.M.Alexander) also went to the Ballarat goldfields, in 1852, but stayed only a short time. His return to Van Diemen's Land was eventful.

On August 5th, 1852, the 'City of Melbourne' sailed from Melbourne for Van Diemen's Land. Built in 1851 in Melbourne this was the first screw steamer in Australia. For this trip the ship carried two hundred and fifty passengers, mainly Tasmanians returning from the Ballarat diggings. It is interesting to note that on the official passenger list there were only fifty four passengers; it was common at the time for people to just go down to the wharf and go aboard, without too many formalities.

Matthias Alexander was one of the two hundred and fifty passengers on this boat, which two days later was struggling in bad weather off the coast of King Island in Bass Strait, a rocky and treacherous coastline which has claimed many ships and hundreds of lives.

The 'City of Melbourne' became grounded, but fortunately all aboard managed to scramble safely ashore. A small boat from the ship was despatched to the not too distant coastline of Van Diemen's Land. After several days, rescue ships arrived with provisions for the by now almost starving passengers, who were then taken to Launceston. Matthias Alexander returned to Table Cape, near Wynyard.

Matthias had married Mary Reading (other spellings include Readen, Redin) in 1838 at Campbell Town, just south of Launceston. There were seven children; the fourth, John, was destined to be the father of Frederick Matthias Alexander. Mary died in 1850, leaving a young family. In 1854 Matthias remarried and there were another seven children from this marriage.

VAN DIEMEN'S LAND 1830'S to 1880'S

Van Diemen's Land, the second colony to be founded in Australia (1803), did not develop large-scale growth as compared with the Australian mainland colonies. The population of 1831, 25,000, did increase, but events both within and outside the colony influenced and shaped its destiny in sometimes unforseen ways.

By the 1830's much of the country in Van Diemen's Land that was easily converted to farming had been taken up by large landowners, free settlers or ex-convicts. There was not enough land to accommodate all those wanting to farm. Stories were told of large tracts of promising farming land in the southernmost parts of New South Wales (i.e., what is now Victoria). A few people moved across from Van Diemen's Land to these areas, which the Surveyor-General (Thomas Mitchell) explored in 1836 and called 'Australia Felix' or 'Australia the Blessed'. An increasing number of people from Van Diemen's Land and other parts of New South Wales came to settle these fertile plains.

The town of Melbourne, on Port Phillip, was officially named in 1837. The whole southernmost part of New South Wales became the fastest developing part of Australia and in 1850 this region was declared by the British Government to be the new and separate Colony of Victoria.

What had been a trickle of settlers from Van Diemen's Land to Victoria in the 1830's and 1840's became an avalanche in the 1850's. The lure of gold discoveries in Victoria from 1851 onwards almost denuded Van Diemen's Land of its able-bodied male population. Particularly on the North Coast of Van Diemen's Land it was relatively simple to board ship and travel across Bass Strait. The journey could be rough and take up to a week, but what was short-term discomfort compared to promises of wealth from the goldfields ? In the long term a number of these hopefuls did return to Tasmania, a few with wealth for their efforts, but many more with disillusionment.

The solid growth of Van Diemen's Land in the 1830's and 1840's was due in large part to the importance of its whaling and shipbuilding industries. This, together with a by now well developed agricultural system, enabled the capital of Van Diemen's Land, Hobart, to have fine public buildings and the well-to-do merchants and pastoralists of the colony to have homes on quite a grand scale, with equally grand accommodation for their horses - all built by convict labour, which was plentiful and cheap.

Transportation of convicts to Van Diemen's Land ceased in 1853. In 1855 a new Constitution was adopted in the colony and the name was changed from Van Diemen's Land to Tasmania. Alongside the shortage of labour in the 1850's there was the need for more workers to assist with maintaining the fast growing export trade to Victoria and New South Wales. The gold boom in these two colonies created demand for goods and it was Tasmanian timber for building, grain and potatoes for food, and other products that caused Tasmanian exports to treble between 1850 and 1855. This thriving export trade did not continue as the mainland of Australia expanded its own food production and timber imports came in from other countries. This meant that prices dropped and also, Victoria brought in a tariff policy that protected its own local industries.

For Tasmania the boom times of the 1850's gave way to stagnation and depression in the 1860's and for most of the 1870's. When British author, Anthony Trollope visited the colony in 1871 he commented, *"it was sad to have visited a British Colony that had seen its best days."* Trollope wrote several books about this visit to Australia and New Zealand.

Agricultural and pastoral activities dominated the flattened economy, and there was little secondary industry. In 1861 the population of Tasmania was 89,000; it increased to only 99,000 by 1870. However by the late 1870's more rapid expansion again took place with the discovery of tin and other metals, and a mining boom began. In 1881 the Tasmanian population was 115,000 rising to 146,000 by 1891. The mining industry developed strongly and became the mainstay of the Tasmanian economy well into the twentieth century.

Once the areas of fertile plains in Tasmania had been settled, new farmers had to take up land which required much hard labour to convert for stock or crops. In the North West of Tasmania (where the three Alexander brothers, Joseph, Matthias and John and their families settled) great forests covered much of the land right down to the rocky coastline.

The clearing of these areas involved felling the trees, burning the debris and sawing the logs into manageable lengths for removal. The bush pioneers worked mainly as individuals, with their families. Initially housing was a bark or slab hut, made more livable as time and money allowed for improvements to be done. Water was usually collected from a nearby creek, or where possible collected in a tank from roof run-off. Food was very basic and as land was cleared, potatoes, other vegetables and grains were planted and farm animals were run in suitable areas.

Rarely did the small farmer need, or afford, hired labour. Mostly the family helped; the wife when she could, apart from her child-raising duties (and families were usually large) and as the children grew, the girls might help with the milking, the boys with the growing of potatoes and other crops. Not infrequently children missed school because they were needed home on the farm for various chores. To survive, the settlers needed to be self-reliant, determined, hard-working, adaptable and with an ability to improvise as a situation demanded.

With years of hard work and doggedness a farmer could consolidate his property and, though many of the first generation of farmers did not live to reap much reward, a number of their descendants were able to prosper. As the early hardships were overcome there was then more time for other things apart from mere survival. Many of the early settlers were illiterate, but there was opportunity for their children to attend school as the education system spread into more remote parts. The schoolmaster or school mistress was an important member of the local community. Local events such as occasional sporting activities, including wood-chopping matches, bush dances and concerts, or a visit to the annual show in a larger town, all combined to make life less of a continuous hard grind and to bring welcome social contact.

For those who did not live in the towns information about current events was brought by the once or twice weekly visits of the mailmen and/or carriers. Some supplies had to be brought to farms and the produce carried away. The delivery of mail was an eagerly awaited event. For many years the state of the roads caused great hardship for those who travelled on them.

In 1832 two British Quakers, James Backhouse and George Walker, travelled in Van Diemen's Land. Part of their comment on road conditions included the following, "*A road in Van Diemen's Land generally means that the trees have been felled and drawn aside, so as to admit the passage of a bullock cart. A large proportion of the way here was one continual slough. My horse was so jaded that I was obliged to alight when between six and seven miles of the Hills, and make the best of my way on foot, often wading up to my knees in mud. The amazing height of the trees, often over two hundred feet, gives to these forests an air of gloomy grandeur. Shaded by these trees the tracks through these forests were always wet.*"

In another section Backhouse writes, "*The ascent of some of the hills was as steep as a horse could climb, and in some places little but bare rocks. Some whitening human bones lay by the side of one of the paths through this dreadful country, in a situation likely for a person exhausted by fatigue to sink down and die. Sometimes we had to lay hold of the manes of our horses, to retain our seats, sometimes to leap over logs in awkward situations, and sometimes it was impracticable to ride. In some places the scrub was so thick that we could not see each other, and when we came upon Table Cape a fern, Pteris esculenta (bracken) was so deep as to obscure us from the view of each other.*

"After ascending to the top of Table Cape (where the Alexanders settled, less than twenty years later) *we passed over some rich, red loam, clothed with luxuriant vegetation. Fern, Prickly Acacia and Musky Aster were so thick as to be passed with difficulty. Tree ferns were numerous and many lofty shrubs were overrun with Macquarie Harbour Vine and White Clematis. Above the shrubs rose stately Stringy-barks and White Gums, attaining to about two hundred feet in height....In the evening we descended a steep place, at the foot of which, on the coast, there was a grassy level, watered by a clear spring. Here we took up our abode for the night, and formed beds of dry fern and branches, under the shelter of a tarpawling and a Honeysuckle tree".*

Travel conditions did not generally improve much in the 1840's, the tracks were quagmires along which the mailmen, carriers and others slogged their way in carts, wagons, by horse or on foot. It was up to the settlers themselves to repair and maintain the tracks in the more remote areas . In some parts where rain was frequent, tracks could easily become impassable for days at a time and crossing the fast flowing rivers was always a challenge. Along the North West coast it was often easier and quicker to travel by boat from one town to another than to go overland.

The big landowners and the wealthy of the two main towns, Hobart and Launceston, had the easier access to the government of Tasmania and so could lobby for funding for their road needs. Road maintenance in smaller towns and outlying areas gradually came under the management of newly formed Municipal Councils and Road Trusts. The Road Trust was elected by the landholders of a road district, this small, elected group then appointed a person to be Collector for the Road Trust of that area. Residents were levied a set amount as contribution to road upkeep which was paid to the Road Trust Collector. Sometimes discussion about allocation of funds became quite heated. One advantage from the improvement of the roads during the 1850's and 1860's was that it became easier for children to travel to school without undue hardship.

Schools in Tasmania were either set up privately by individuals or church denominations, or were government run. Obviously standards would vary depending on the talent of each teacher. In 1854 the Governor of Tasmania appointed Thomas Arnold as School Inspector for the Colony. He was the son of Thomas Arnold, who was a highly respected and leading reformer of education in England and who held with distinction the Headmastership of Rugby School from 1828 to 1842. Another son was Matthew Arnold, educationist and poet. Both Thomas Arnold (senior) and Matthew

Arnold had strong links with Oxford University. So Tasmania was fortunate to have Thomas Arnold (junior) as School Inspector, a man who came from such a distinguished scholastic background.

In December 1854 Thomas Arnold, in a Report to the Tasmanian Board of Education, spoke on various aspects of what he had found when visiting schools in most of the settled areas of the Colony. With regards to teachers the Report states, *"There has been no lack of applications during the half-year from persons desirous of employment as schoolmasters; but few of the applicants, I am sorry to say, have been possessed of real professional qualifications. The preliminary examination required of candidates by the Board - the first of the kind, I believe, attempted in the Australian Colonies - has had an excellent effect"*. In order to develop a standard of teaching the Board brought a number of trained Teachers from overseas to teach in Tasmania.

Another section of this December 1854 Report states, *"Public Education in this Colony has much to contend with in the indifference with which the subject is frequently regarded. No plea is thought too trifling to excuse a child's absence from School"*. However interest in education did increase. In 1854 the Colony had fifty schools and an enrolment of 2,734 children, in 1855 there were sixty three schools and an enrolment of 3,377 children. A healthy increase. The main subjects taught were Reading, Writing, Arithmetic, Geography, Grammar and History. In regard to the ages of the children attending school, tables show the percentages were on a par with education in Great Britain at the time (1855).

The Education Report by Mr.Stephens for 1858 for the northern part of Tasmania indicates some difficulties, *"for raising local contributions to meet the grant from the General Revenue for building purposes, and the want of a regular supply of qualified and experienced Teachers"*. There were not only monetary problems with regard to establishing schools. *"In many places it is impossible to define, with any certainty, the future centres of population, and consequently undesirable to erect permanent School-houses"*. To overcome this difficulty it was suggested that some itinerant teachers be employed who could use whatever temporary accommodation was available as a schoolroom.

The 1858 Report made special reference to conditions on the North West coast of Tasmania, *" The settlers along the North-west Coast are, for the most part, in narrow circumstances, - the recent fall in the price of timber and potatoes, their staple article of export, having proved a serious calamity to men who depended on them almost solely for subsistence. In no other part of the world, probably, are there such formidable obstacles to the clearing and cultivation of land as here beset the settler of small capital, while the difficulties to be encountered in crossing dangerous tidal rivers, and travers-*

ing forests, where the track, seldom well defined, is in many places entirely obliterated by the rapid growth of underwood, check all free intercommunication and isolate him almost completely from the notice and sympathy of settled civilisation".

By 1860, though the number of children enrolled in the Government Schools had increased, there was also the feeling that education could be made more appropriate for the needs of the Colony. Three probable causes of indifference to Education by those people who did not encourage their children to attend school were listed as follows in the 1860 Education Board Report:

"1. The isolation of many families in the bush, where even a migratory Master can hardly reach them. This is, I fear, irremediable.

2. The objection to the Schools as more or less proceeding from or connected with the Government. This almost instinctive aversion is very powerful with the still considerable section of the people who have been prisoners. They have an antipathy to the Schools because Government supports them.

3. Above all, in a country where manual labour suffices for the necessaries and many of the comforts of life, a large number, uneducated themselves, cannot see the use of Education for their children. This is an evil which no external measures can cure, but which must cure itself through the action of the Schools themselves. As the parents die off, their children, better trained, will offer no such obstacles; and the lapse of time may be trusted to remedy an evil which no Legislative measures can reach".

The 1860 Report continues, *"It must be always borne in mind, in attempting to carry out any general system of Education in Tasmania, that, from the circumstances of the settlement of the Colony, uniformity cannot be obtained, and if obtained would be undesirable. Each district, and almost each separate school, requires a modification to suit its particular circumstances. ..The State of Tasmania differs widely from that of any of the United Kingdom or States of America. The Tasmanian school system, however, is framed exclusively upon the model of the National Schools at home, and especially those in use under the National Board of Education in Ireland".*

The 1862 Report by the Northern Board of Education in Tasmania refers to the fact that, *"We have felt it necessary to place somewhat stringent restrictions upon the employment of Pupil Teachers, partly on account of the necessity of economising the funds placed at our disposal, but also because it appeared undesirable that any but those who gave fair promise of ultimately becoming useful as Teachers should be employed in Schools at the public expense".*

This system of appointing a Pupil Teacher, called a Monitor, was a useful one, especially where in a one-teacher school, the teacher had to cope with a number of children of varied age and learning abilities. F.M.Alexander was appointed a school Monitor in the 1880's in Wynyard.

The standard of teacher qualifications was a constant concern of School Inspectors so it was with a degree of satisfaction that the following appeared in the 1870 Education Report, *"The end of the year was marked by an event which ought not to be passed over without notice - the first general examination of Teachers that has ever been held in Tasmania.*
......As the chief object of the scheme of classification is to induce Teachers to make themselves thoroughly qualified for their profession, for which few have been systematically trained, it is indispensable that a reasonably high standard both of practical and theoretical skill be required, and that it be clearly shown that a Certificate of Merit is really what its name imports".

The 1871 Education Report has further comment re teachers; *"The result of the last general Examination of Teachers shows that the difficulty of obtaining a Certificate of Merit has been somewhat underrated by candidates for promotion. The scheme of classification was expressly designed to make the increase of salary contingent upon the exhibition of practical skill combined with theoretical knowledge, and the only defect that has hitherto become apparent is its tendency to give to the young Teachers who have but recently emerged from a state of pupilage an undue advantage over those who are unaccustomed to the routine of Examinations, though possessing those higher qualifications which are gained by experience alone."* Also noted is, *"the absence of any adequate provision for the training of Teachers".*

The observations about the skills needed to be a teacher are interesting, as in 1879 Mr.Robert Robertson (F.M. Alexander's teacher) was appointed Teacher at the Wynyard School, mainly because of the special qualities he showed for teaching, not because of any formal teaching qualifications.

The life of a School Inspector was not an easy one. The 1873 General Report on Education notes the following, *"The actual business of travelling consumes a large portion of my time, and the year's work, imperfect as it is, has not been accomplished without much personal sacrifice of private time and money, no means having been spared that would enable me at any time to do two days' work in one. The hardships and privations often encountered on bush journeys in bad weather are necessary accompaniments of an Inspector's life, and must be accepted as a matter of course".*

Again, in the 1875 Report, "*An Inspector's profession is chiefly to be learned by experience, and personal qualifications are those which are most required. He ought to have a practical knowledge of teaching and school management, but above all things it is essential that he shall have had such a liberal up-bringing as will enable him to judge fairly and treat with respect the views which may happen to differ from his own, and to understand that all Teachers are not intended to work in exactly the same groove. An aptitude for bush travelling, and an unlimited capacity for roughing it, are very necessary qualifications for Inspectors, though the facilities for travelling are much improved, and they will be exempt from the necessity of swimming unfordable rivers, which used formerly to be a common incident of my North Coast journeys*".

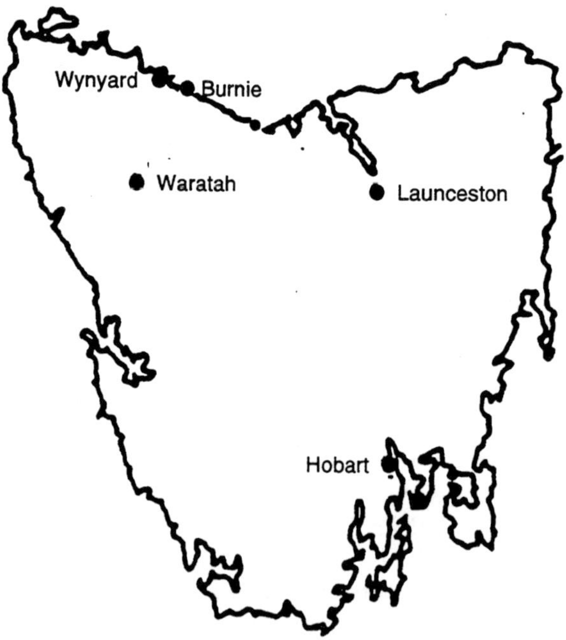

Tasmania

F.M. ALEXANDER WYNYARD AND WARATAH

The Alexanders

Exploration of the thickly forested land comprising most of the North West coast of Tasmania had begun in the 1820's. From the point of view of settlement the reports were not encouraging, one report stated the region *"is quite impenetrable and totally uninhabitable"*. But settlement of parts of the region did begin slowly. In 1841 a family settled at Table Cape, very close to where Wynyard now is, and cleared and farmed the rich, red loam, in almost complete isolation.

In 1850 the two Alexander brothers, Joseph and Matthias, began the first settlement on the west side of the Inglis River, on the opposite side to where the town of Wynyard is now situated. The younger brother John joined them in the mid 1850's after his success at the Ballarat goldfields. A small community developed here, called Alexandria. The Alexander families ran a hotel, opened a store, had a schooner, the Alexander, built for produce and timber trading, and they cleared and farmed a large area of nearby Table Cape. By the 1860's the small village of Alexandria declined as the township of Wynyard on the opposite side of the Inglis River grew. Members of the Alexander families continued to farm the Table Cape area for many years.

Today, the region supports a diverse economy based on agricultural produce, mining, and timber from the large forests, used as building materials and (the poorer cuts) as pulp for paper manufacture. The conditions of life in the rich agricultural areas with their clearly fenced, lush pastures running top quality dairy herds, bounteous crops sown in well ordered fashion using the latest highly mechanised farm machinery, attractive farm houses and an organised road system are in total contrast to the scene with which the pioneers would have been familiar.

Then, huge trees had to be felled and got rid of. One way, if you were by the edge of a cliff-top, was to roll the logs over the cliffs to crash into the sea below; as well as the enormous eucalypts, there were many other species of trees and smaller undergrowth, all to be cleared, and the rich soil prepared for crops. This was done by hand with only very basic tools and the help of bullock teams. Once the produce was harvested, getting it to town to sell involved man and beast (horse or bullock) toiling along the rough bush tracks.

Much of the original natural beauty of this region is still the same today: magnificent stands of forest, the wild mountainous country with swift flowing rivers through deep gorges covered with dense scrub. The tallest mountains attain a height of over 5,000 feet. Some of the more isolated mountains, though of lesser height, are equally spectacular and can be seen outlined starkly on the horizon from various points along the coastline.

The lighthouse on Table Cape, built in 1885, still stands, etched against the skyline on the edge of a cliff two hundred metres above sea level. Nearby Fossil Bluff, close to Wynyard, is a remarkable geological formation, one hundred feet high, composed mostly of sea shells. Here, the oldest fossil marsupial ever found was unearthed .

This then is the land where the Alexander brothers, Joseph, Matthias and John settled and brought up their families. Matthias remarried in 1854, after the death of his first wife in 1850. The children from the first marriage included a son, John. When he grew up he became a blacksmith. In 1866 he married Betsey Brown at the nearby town of Somerset. They lived up on Table Cape, where they raised a large family. Their eldest son was :

Frederick Matthias Alexander 1869 - 1955

Frederick Matthias Alexander was born on January 20th, 1869. His schooling took place in Wynyard, which by the 1870's had a population of about two hundred people. The boundaries of the town itself and outlying areas were not clear and some degree of population change was continuous. Early school records for the area show that the name Alexander was on school rolls, so when FM went to the Wynyard school in the 1870's he was yet another Alexander to be part of the local school community.

The present Wynyard Public School (run under the State Education system) began in 1871 with an enrolment of twenty-nine children. The second headmaster, Mr.Robert Robertson, was appointed in 1879 and was in charge there until 1886. So during his headship he would have been the school teacher who influenced the young F.M. Alexander.

Robert Robertson was born in March 1854 in Stirling, Scotland. He trained and worked as a law clerk, then emigrated to Tasmania in 1875. In 1876 he applied to be a teacher in the Tasmanian State Education system. He satisfactorily passed the examination for the teaching of class subjects and was accepted as a teacher though he had had no previous practical experience. His report stated that, *"Robert Robertson appears to possess some of the best natural qualifications for the office of teacher."*

After teaching at the Wynyard school from 1879 to 1886, Robert Robertson took leave from March to November 1886 and apparently returned to England. On his return to Tasmania he asked to be reappointed to Wynyard; this was not possible, and he was appointed to teach at Hamilton, where he died in 1888, aged thirty-four years. He left a wife and young family.

Frederick Matthias Alexander must have made good progress at school because in December 1883, aged fourteen years, he was appointed to be a paid Monitor at the Wynyard school, remaining in that position until August 1885. The position of paid Monitor meant an older pupil would be given duties to carry out under the head teacher. It is said that FM's teacher, Robert Robertson, was the one who encouraged and developed the lad's love of literature, especially poetry and Shakespeare.

About this time FM visited Waratah, fifty miles inland from the coast, and the site of what was for a time, the richest tin mine in the world, Mt.Bischoff. This visit led to change in FM's life, change which gave opportunities to explore an ever widening variety of experience. As a result of the visit FM was offered a job with the Mt. Bischoff Mining Company as a junior accountant. He accepted.

Waratah - Mt Bischoff

The ease with which mining companies of today can fly in men and equipment to remote areas by plane or helicopter is in stark contrast to how prospectors and miners worked last century. The West coast of Tasmania has some of the most impenetrable forest, and a wet climate. As well as the immense trees, some of which, when fallen, make obstacles of great difficulty, there are smaller trees, shrubs and ferns, and worst of all the horizontal scrub. This consists of certain types of small trees that grow a few feet then bend horizontally, and as the branches continue to grow they intertwine so that the resulting foliage is in some places impossible to penetrate.

Add to this the mountainous nature of the terrain, the steep slopes leading down to gorges with swift flowing rivers, and a climate which can change within a few hours from warmth and sunshine to mists, rain and even snow, is it any wonder that it was only the most hardy prospectors who would attempt to traverse these regions in an endeavour to unlock the secrets of the mineral wealth which lay hidden beneath the surface of this wild, mysterious, challenging land.

The intermittent attempts by the early explorers to map the West coast gave way in the 1870's and 80's to more frequent visits to the area by explorer-prospectors who, as they criss-crossed the country, were able to fill in the

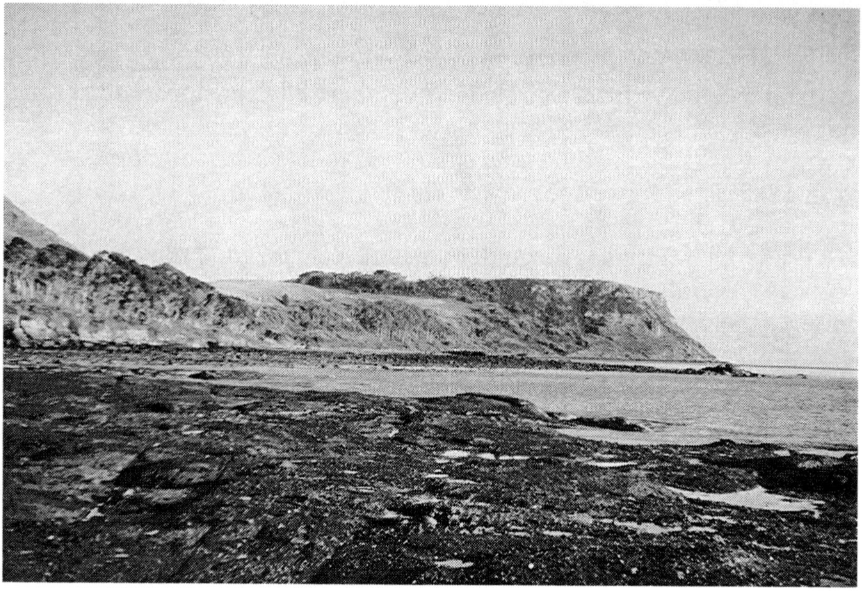

View from Fossil Beach towards Table Cape

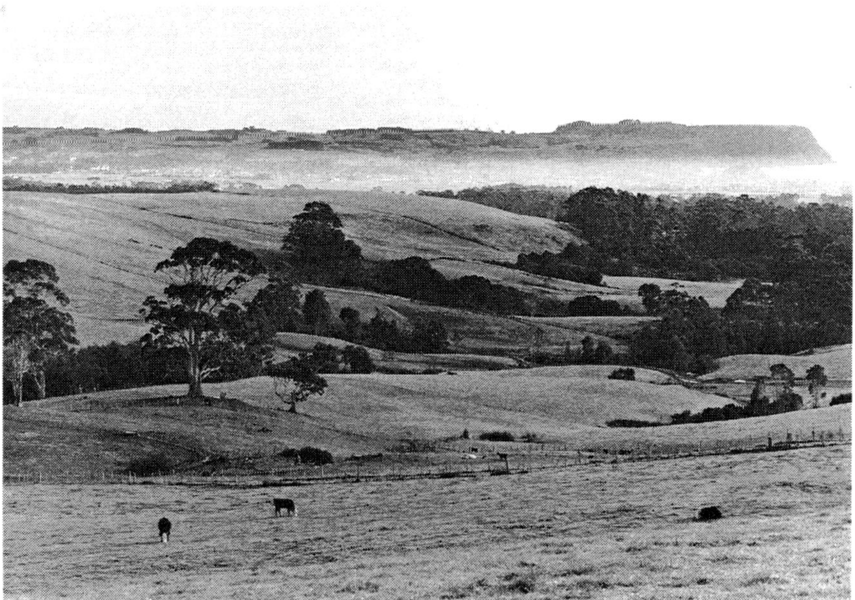

General view, Wynyard and Table Cape (Courtesy of Margaret Long)

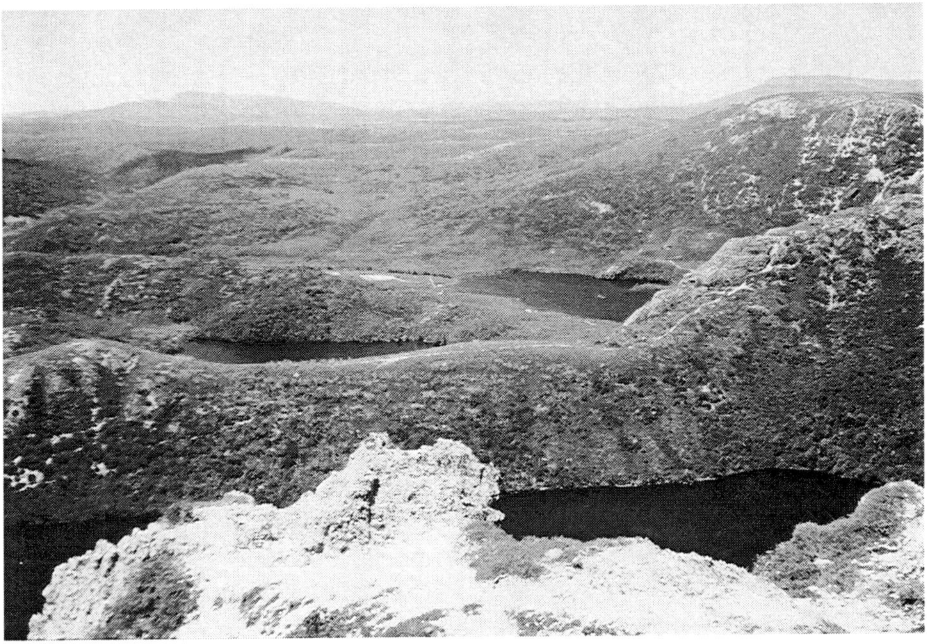

Mountainous Range, Western Tasmania

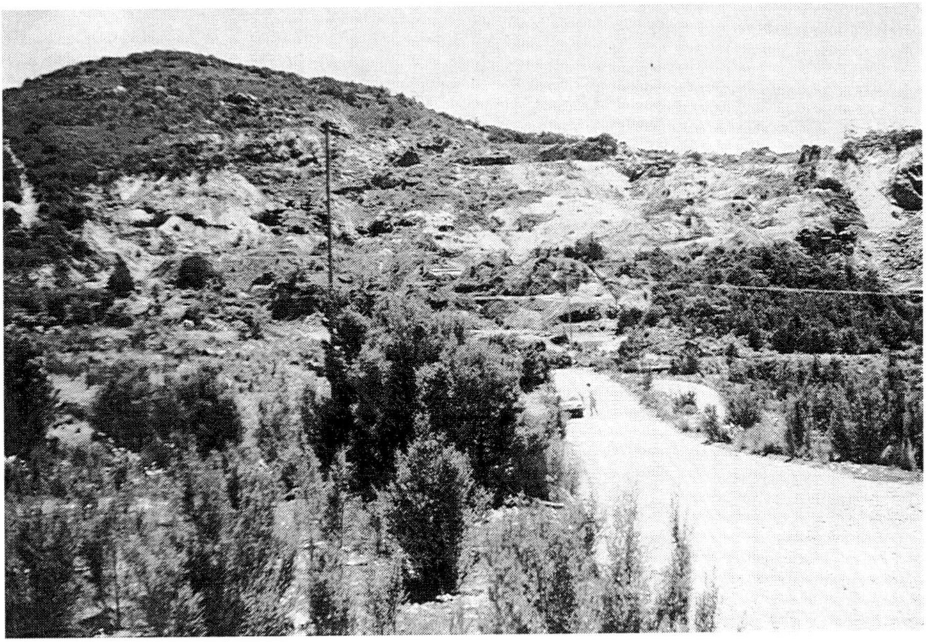

Part of Mt Bischoff today

detail of the region. One of the most experienced and persevering of these men was James Smith, who had begun his exploring in the 1850's and was to continue to do so for many decades. He died in 1897.

James Smith was a widely read, mostly self-educated man with knowledge on many subjects. He became known as 'Philosopher' Smith. He owned land not far from Ulverstone, on the coast, but farming was secondary to his main mission, that of prospecting. 'Philosopher' Smith made numerous finds of metals but his most outstanding discovery in 1871was that of tin at Mt.Bischoff.

Mining began at the Mt.Bischoff Tin Mine in 1872, but major progress came later when the mine was managed by Mr.H.W.F.Kayser. Appointed as Mine Manager in 1875 he held the position for over thirty years. His thorough scientific training in Germany and practical mining experience in many places, including a number of years in Victoria, made him an excellent choice for the job of managing a mine which at one stage dominated the world tin market and was the richest tin mine in the world.

The town of Waratah which grew alongside the mine was initially just a camp; by 1881 there was a population of eight hundred and seventy four people, which peaked at 5,000 in the heyday of the town then declined rapidly as mining towns are wont to do once the purpose for their existence, the mineral resource, is gone. However as the output from the Mt.Bischoff Tin Mine started to decline, (after operating for over fifty years,) rich mineral deposits were found in other areas of the West coast and still today there is both mining and mineral exploration in the region.

Once mining began at Mt.Bischoff in 1872 the ore had to be got to the coast at Burnie (then called Emu Bay) for shipment to Melbourne where it was smelted. At first cartage from the mine was by bullock teams over the very rough tracks, a cumbersome, time-consuming and often unreliable method of transport. As well, machinery and goods had to be brought to the mine from Burnie. There was an obvious need for transport operations to be more efficient.

A decision was made in 1875 by the Van Diemen's Land Company, a large pastoral and investment Company in Tasmania (founded 1825 and still in existence), to build a wooden tramway from Burnie jetty to the Mt.Bischoff Mine, a distance of forty-eight miles. The Herculean task of constructing this tramway took just over three years, across most difficult terrain and with frequent halts because of inclement weather, particularly in winter. From the coast at Burnie the gradient inland for the tramway track had to rise to an elevation of 2,000 feet by the time it reached the outlying area of Waratah.

This tramway journey from Burnie to three miles outside of the Mt.Bischoff Mine and Waratah could take seven or eight hours, or longer if there were difficulties, such as bad weather (because of disagreements the tramway track was not fully completed). Travel was not pleasant, both passengers and goods were put in uncovered trolleys placed on the wooden rails and pulled by horses, but at least the passenger trolleys were provided with benches to sit on. The ride certainly would have been quite bumpy.

As both passenger and goods traffic increased for this line, it became obvious that a more efficient system of transport was needed. Work was begun in 1883 and completed in 1884 to convert the tramway to a steam railway line. The wooden rails had to be changed to steel rails and locomotives used to haul the carriages. Rolling stock for the project arrived from England in July 1883, at the Port of Burnie.

At the time, port facilities for unloading were very basic, and larger ships such as the two that brought the railway rolling stock, including two locomotives, from England, could not tie up at the jetty. So the ships dropped anchor in the bay and small craft were used to transfer all the equipment ashore, a process which took five months, and was made difficult by often rough seas and the size and weight of the equipment. The actual railway line right into Waratah was completed and in operation by July 1884.

As improvements were made, the first regular service began in March 1885; the journey from Burnie to Waratah now took half the time previously taken by the tramways, and this three and a half hours travel time included several intermediate stops. The passenger train carriages were certainly more comfortable than the open trolleys of the tramway, the ride was smoother but there was certainly room for improvement in the safety area.

The locomotives and carriages had been bought after rejection by the Indian State Railways so upgrading of the equipment became a necessity. Though there were no fatal accidents, the then Chief Agent of the VDL Company which had built both the tramway and the railway line wrote at the time of the railway opening (1884), *"It is not a pleasing sensation on watching a train leaving the station to know that it may be the cause before it returns of getting one imprisoned for manslaughter"*.

F.M. Alexander and Waratah

So the town in which F.M.Alexander came to live, in 1885, had a new railway link to Burnie; it had an electric telegraph, a facility which had come to the North West region in the mid 1870's, and allowed farmers to make quicker decisions about the marketing of their agricultural produce; it had a population of 2,500 - no doubt diverse as mining towns are wont to be; it had much of the organisational resources that provide people with the necessary social, cultural and community conditions for a reasonably well-ordered life. These resources included post office, bank, six large general stores, three hotels, a temperance hotel, schools, hospital, dentist and Mechanics Institute.

The Mechanics Institute had a library of over 2,000 books; a wide range of British and Colonial newspapers, magazines,etc.; there was a large hall capable of accommodating three hundred people and equipped with stage, scenery, dressing rooms etc.; also a reading-room, games room and museum of mineral collections. In 1885 the annual subscription was twelve shillings. A Mechanics Institute was a multi-purpose place, it was the cultural heart of a town.

The idea for the formation of Mechanics Institutes' started in Scotland in the early 1800's with classes being organised to educate working-men and give instruction in various trades. The scheme grew, spread to England and broadened its aim to encompass general adult education. The first Mechanics Institute in Australia was founded in Hobart in 1827. Subsequently Mechanics Institutes were established in the other Australian Colonies; by 1870 New South Wales alone had nearly seventy. Sometimes the name used was Schools of Arts. As well as providing library facilities, the Mechanics Institute would be the venue for lectures on a wide range of subjects and other such educational or cultural activities as the local populace wanted.

Around Waratah there was wilderness - mountains, dense forest, large rocky outcrops, deep gorges and fast flowing rivers. During the last part of the 1800's explorer - prospectors continued to traverse the more remote parts, and to find worthwhile and sometimes rich deposits of various metals. These finds led to new mining towns being established and the decline of Waratah in the early part of the 20th century. Today Waratah's population is about four hundred with here and there reminders of the town's historic past.

F.M.Alexander lived in Waratah for three years. As well as his job as a junior accountant at the Mt.Bischoff Tin Mine he later obtained the position as Collector for the local Road Trust. The monies levied by these Trusts were used to upgrade the sometimes deplorable state of the roads in the local area.

Alexander was seventeen years old when he was appointed to this responsible job and his appointment indicates the high regard there must have been for his capabilities. The letter of appointment in 1886 includes the following, *"Before you enter upon the duties it will be necessary for you to hand me* (the Chairman of the Waratah Road Trust) *a written Bond to the amount of one hundred pounds, yourself in fifty pounds and two respectable persons in the sums of twenty five pounds each, I enclose a copy of Bond for your guidance".* In those days a bond of one hundred pounds would have been a large amount.

The role of Mine Manager in a mining town is a powerful one, not only with regard to mine matters but also in connection with the well-being of the miners' families and the general standards of the town. Mr.H.W.F.Kayser (1833 - 1919) was appointed Mine Manager in 1875 and retired in 1898. He came from Germany to Australia in 1853, worked as a miner, mine manager, and farmer , mainly in Victoria, then moved to the Mt.Bischoff Mine in Tasmania as Manager in 1875. Mr.Kayser cared for the welfare of the people, he had good houses built, and in 1883 the town and mine were lit by the use of hydro-electricity, a first in an Australian industrial plant. He held a number of official positions in Waratah, including being on the Board of the Road Trust. Mr. Kayser certainly would have had contact with the young FM Alexander and his influence would have been beneficial.

During his three years in Waratah (1885 - 1888) FM*, apart from his work, took the opportunity to develop his interests in the arts. He did some violin study but his main hobby was taking part in amateur dramatic performances. There was scope for giving entertainments to the locals, by the locals, and as well there were performances by visiting artists. So isolated towns did not lack for creative, artistic activities and stimulus.

However after three years FM was thinking of broader horizons where he could explore, learn and be challenged. There were many members of the Alexander families, some with fascinating stories to tell. No doubt as a lad growing up in Wynyard, FM would have been aware of his heritage. He did not know his grandfather, Matthias, who died in 1865, but the two brothers of Matthias lived in the Wynyard area until 1878 (Joseph) and 1898 (John) respectively. The adventurous life of John Alexander in going to the Californian goldfields, then having success at the Ballarat goldfields in Victoria would have been a talked-of part of the family history. With relatives living in Melbourne and, no doubt, news about events in this wealthy, progressive, culturally lively city reaching across Bass Strait to Tasmania, is it any wonder that FM was drawn to thoughts of travel, to finding out for himself what Marvellous Melbourne had to offer?

* The initials FM will be used for F.M.Alexander.

MARVELLOUS MELBOURNE

Frederick Matthias Alexander came to Melbourne in the late 1880's when the city was on the crest of a wave. It had fine public buildings, business was booming, the arts were well established, Melbourne was justifiably in good spirits and somewhat pleased with itself. FM had high hopes of developing his dramatic and other artistic abilities, with the ultimate goal of becoming a professional. However, dreams take time to be transformed into realities. After soaking himself in the richness of Melbourne cultural life for a few months, FM took decisions regarding his future that allowed him to make a living and take the necessary steps towards a career as reciter and actor.

The great impetus for Australia's meteoric growth in the 1850's was due to gold. Exports of the precious metal during this decade were worth about eight million pounds annually. It overtook wool as the main Australian export. From about the 1870's the quantity of found gold slowly declined, and wool and other products headed the export stakes. Victoria had had the lion's share of the gold discoveries for thirty years (1850's to 1880's) and the largest population increase, so the capital, Melbourne, naturally became the financial 'capital' of Australia.

In 1885 a visiting British journalist, George Sala, wrote of Melbourne that there were fine thoroughfares; variety of transport; splendid cathedrals and other places of worship; imposing public buildings such as the Town Hall, General Post Office, a dignified Government House residence for Her Majesty's (Queen Victoria's) representative, a grand Exhibition Building (built for the 1880 Melbourne International Exhibition) and what would be, when finished, impressive Houses of Parliament; a splendid University; big banks and insurance buildings of palatial design; plus theatres, schools, hospitals, hotels, etc; many parks, gardens and recreation grounds. In short, Melbourne could, and did, feel flushed with pride at the rapid development that changed it from the 'Canvas Town' of the 1850's (population 23,000 in 1852) to the Melbourne of the 1880's (population 290,000 in 1880). This George Sala called Marvellous Melbourne.

The decade of the 1880's saw the population of Melbourne nearly double, by 1890 it was 491,000. The growth of Sydney, the capital of the mother-colony of New South Wales, had been slower, reaching 384,000 by 1890. Subsequently, in the last decade of the century, New South Wales with its larger land mass and greater range of natural resources, again achieved population supremacy. In the period of the 1880's with Melbourne's rapid growth there was increased secondary industry; the commercial heart of the city expanded; there was not only one Stock Exchange, but six in operation, plus a number of banks which had cheques to a total value of eighty-seven million pounds in the first half of 1887, and to the total value of one hundred and sixty-five million in the first half of 1888; and there was the land boom, with speculators increasingly gambling with land sales.

In 1887 the Golden Jubilee of Queen Victoria was enthusiastically celebrated. On the actual date, June 20th, there was a night of festivity in the city attended by an estimated crowd of 200,000 people, who came to admire the artificial stars, the crowns and mottos of the illuminations and the fine facades of the public buildings, all picked out in the new-fangled electric light.

In 1888, the boom year of the boom decade, Melbourne celebrated Australia's Centenary as part of the British Empire by holding a grandiose Centennial Exhibition in the Exhibition Building. These flourishing times and the extravagant, often reckless way of life, could not continue. The 1880's was life in the fast lane, the 1890's was learning to come to terms with changes that forced people to be more realistic about what was possible and what was not. A combination of circumstances and events, both within and outside Victoria, brought the once optimistic, brash, swaggering attitude of endless optimism to one of hopelessness, despair and soul-searching; an experience from which Melbourne recovered slowly.

For Victoria, the 1890's saw a reduction of the flow of British capital into the Colony; a substantial drop in the prices that exports such as wool and wheat had brought on the overseas markets; there was industrial unrest, businesses collapsed, unemployment grew, many people left Victoria to go to the newly discovered goldfields in Western Australia; people who had speculated in shares or land sales, either for themselves, or worse, on behalf of others, had to face their creditors; and there was a run on the banks and building societies - a number of which went under. Land boom turned to land bust, people who had made fortunes through business ventures became paupers overnight.

The whole of Australia was affected by these times of hardship and economic depression, but by the end of the century recovery and confidence were well restored. The 1890's crash hit Victoria most severely. However the fabric of life did develop new patterns and though for a time life was hard, the artistic life of the colony, its theatre, music and art, continued to evolve and grow.

It was Melbourne's cultural life that had attracted FM Alexander in the late 1880's. The mainstream of theatre, music, art and literature were lively and diversified. Then there were the other, none-the-less important, aspects of cultural and social life, such as the clubs, (formed, and sometimes disbanded, after a short life), which covered many interests; lectures, too, on diverse topics, featured strongly.

From its beginnings in 1788 as a British colony, Australia soon started to develop entertainments of various types which, over about a fifty year span, included Shakespeare, opera, pantomime, burlesque and circus. Many of the performances were of indifferent standard and often given under difficult conditions that included somewhat rowdy audience behaviour, though the performers, on the other side of the stage, were not slow, on occasion, to retaliate.

The gold rush era of the 1850's saw rapid growth of colonial theatre; increased finance was available, and the gold rush provided playwrights with a wealth of material, and emotional range from ecstasy to despair. There was much coming and going of performers between England, America and Australia, and theatre building commenced in earnest.

George Coppin (1819-1906) was for several decades one of the most influential theatre people in Australia. In December 1892, Table Talk (Melbourne Weekly) gave a lengthy profile of his life, the following are extracts: *"Mr Coppin was born on April 8, 1819, and went on the English stage at a very early age. He soon made his mark in the line of low comedy, of which he subsequently became such a complete master. He arrived in Sydney in March, 1843, being the first English star of any repute who accepted an Australian engagement."*

After Sydney Coppin went to Tasmania thence to Melbourne, *"where he appeared as manager and actor for the first time at the Queen's Theatre on June 21, 1845, more than 47 years ago. From that date to the present Mr.Coppin has been intimately associated with the Melbourne stage, though at intervals he has managed theatres in other colonies."*

After a variety of experiences in Australia he returned to England in 1854, played many principal theatres and engaged artists for new productions in Australia. Coppin also, *"had a portable iron theatre built to his order in Manchester for erection in Melbourne, an experiment which illustrates, as much as any other part of his various ventures, the unbounded enterprise of the man."*

Once back in Melbourne George Coppin's busy life involved performance, management and theatre building. *"On June 11, 1856, he inaugurated the first grand opera season ever introduced into the Australian colonies, and this was followed by a season of English opera."*

Over the years, alongside all his entrepeneurial activities George Coppin *"always did immense service as an actor"* performing for the last time in Melbourne in 1881. *"For several years past he has taken an active part in political affairs, and as a member of Parliament he has done the State great service. Whilst a member of the Legislative Assembly Mr. Coppin introduced and carried the Post Office Savings Banks Bill, and the "Torrens Act" for the transfer of real property, two measures which have proved of the utmost utility to the public. Since his election to the Upper House of the Legislature Mr. Coppin has been a keen critic of all measures brought before the Council. It is, however, as a theatrical manager and actor that his work will be most remembered when the events of the last half century have passed into history, and it is in this double capacity that he is principally entitled to the everlasting gratitude of the present and future generations of Victoria."*

Another giant of theatre life in Australia for many decades was J.C.Williamson (b 1845, America - d 1913, France).He arrived in Melbourne in 1874 to star in the play Struck Oil which did indeed strike it rich financially, for both J.C.Williamson and his wife. As with Coppin, Australia became the home for the Williamsons. J.C.Williamson not only fulfilled acting engagements himself, but became theatre manager and entrepreneur, with such success, that by 1900, "The Firm" (as the J.C.Williamson organisation was known) had a near monopolistic position in professional theatre management. It was J.C.Williamson, and Garner and Co. who brought to Australia the legendary French actress Sarah Bernhardt. Her visit in 1891, to Melbourne, Adelaide and Sydney with a complete French company created enormous public interest, and adulation.

Theatre buildings in the two main capital cities, Sydney and Melbourne, varied greatly in their grandeur, and otherwise. In the latter half of the 1800's theatre patrons expected more comfort, and some theatres provided most lavish surroundings; whilst the demands of some plays created the need for ever more wondrous scenery and the development of intricate stage machinery. That nightmare for a theatre owner, a theatre fire, happened all too often, though fortunately with minimal loss of life; but did result in government tightening fire-proofing regulations, and insisting on better exit facilities. The major theatres of Sydney and Melbourne could accommodate anything from 2,000 to 3,000 people, so should there be any emergency, quick escape routes were certainly needed. This era also saw the introduction of electric light to replace gaslight, which, as one actor lamented, cast a harsher light than the soft glow of gaslight.

Literary magazines and periodicals were an integral part of Australian literature. Melbourne from its beginnings, (late 1830's) to the end of that century produced almost two hundred such journals. Some had short lives. But whether via journals or the main daily newspapers (of which there were three) the drama, music, literary and art critics were usually given ample space to report their findings and opinions. It is from sources such as these that we today can gain some insight into the cultural life of a bygone era.

The Australian population of last century was mainly of British origin. Once the pioneering days were over and the frenzy of the early gold fever of the 1850's subsided, it was natural that at least some of the populace would give consideration to intellectual and artistic pursuits without necessarily wanting to become professional in these areas. The educated, cultivated amateur who is willing to devote time, and often money, to cultural endeavours, is a necessary part of society. People who emigrated from England or other countries, brought past cultural associations which became tinged with nostalgia as time further distanced them from their homeland.

James Smith (1820 - 1910) is a good example of the British emigrant who maintained cultural links with the Old Country through the varied activities which involved him during his time in Melbourne, from 1854 until his death there in 1910. His profession was that of journalist and critic, and he was on the staff of The Argus (a Melbourne daily) for most of his journalistic career. The main organisations with which James Smith became associated at some time or another included the Garrick Club, Victorian Society of Fine Arts, Press Cricket Club, Royal Society, Garibaldi Memorial Fund, Yorick Club, Athenaeum Club, Public Library, French Literary Club, Working Men's Club, Caxton Fund (to celebrate the fourth centenary of the first printing in the English language by William Caxton in 1471), Dante Society, Melbourne Elocution Society, Melbourne Shakespeare Society and Alliance Francaise. James Smith was often a founding member of these groups and, as well, a committee member of a number of them. The last three named Societies merit explanation.

The Melbourne Elocution Society was founded in 1863. Little is known of its existence, though it lasted for at least twenty years. The topic of elocution was a high priority in the colonies; over the years one can find spirited references to the need for clear speech. As the number of native-born Australians increased, there was reference to the colonial accent (or Australian twang) as though it was something that should be modified, or got rid of. Elocutionists were much sought-after, particularly by those in professions where public speaking was a necessity. In the schools, the study of elocution was treated as a regular subject. In a Speech Day Report of 1902 Miss Morris, the Headmistress of Melbourne Church of England Girls Grammar School, a leading girls school in Melbourne, noted that the examiner in elocution, " *approved particularly of the reading of the juniors and noticed a commendable absence of that very common and disagreeable colonial twang which is usual amongst the young people of the State*".

The clergy were conscious of the need for good speech delivery. The Baptist Theological College in Melbourne engaged an elocutionist to work with the students for the ministry. The Southern Baptist Newspaper, March 16th, 1899, comments on this matter, " *Our conviction is that in training students more heed should be given to the cultivation of the powers of speech. Much valuable cargo is wrecked on the harbour-bar of imperfect modes of speech. The mouthing, artificial, monotonous, see-saw style of some men makes unacceptable to ordinary folks matter of large worth. A teacher of rhetoric is a necessary addition to the staff of every college".*

As well as theatre of the type requiring a large company of performers, elaborate scenery and usually plenty of space to accommodate the audience, there were other styles of entertainment, including the elocutionary recital. The main artist, who would recite a number of contrasting pieces, poems (humorous and pathetic) and extracts from Shakespeare, Charles Dickens or others, would have associate artists on the programme. These could include other actors or actresses, a singer and one or more instrumentalists.

The following is an extract from an interview, *"A Chat about Elocution with Mr.Lawrence Campbell"*, done by a reporter from the Sydney Daily Telegraph, reprinted in the North West Post, Devonport (Tasmania) on July 28th, 1894. Mr.Campbell is described as a clever young English elocutionist who has recently come to live in Sydney.

"There are two sides to every question", said Mr.Campbell, " *and there are two sides to elocution. There is the mechanical side involving a study of articulation, enunciation, emphasis, and grammatical pauses; and there is the sentimental side, implying considerations of tone, pitch, inflection, rhetorical pauses, facial expression and gesture. A student with any aptitude will grasp the principles upon which the mechanical branch of the art is based in the course of six months; but he will want at least three years training before he is able to apply them successfully. Even then success will depend upon laborious daily practice. The teacher's first object is to see that every syllable is clearly articulated and that one word is spoken distinctly before the next word is begun. Then comes the necessity for correct accentuation, and, lastly, for due emphasis. What articulation is to the syllable and accentuation to the word, emphasis is to the sentence.*

"Coming to the sentimental side of the art, what could appear more easy than the uplifting of a hand or the outgoing of a foot? What more simply natural than that the movement of the limbs should keep pace with the movement of the theme? Yet in point of fact gesticulation forms one of the most serious difficulties to be encountered by the student...

"Then there is an important difference between classic gesture and comedy gesture" continued Mr.Campbell. *"In classic gesture all arm movements are formed in sweeping curves from the shoulder; in comedy gesture they are light and flippant depending chiefly upon the flexibility of the wrist... Elocution on the platform is one thing"*, says Mr.Campbell, *"and elocution on the stage quite another thing, the result being that very few actors make good elocutionists and very few elocutionists good actors. The actor"*, he points out, *"is accustomed to rely, to a large extent, upon stage accessories, whilst the elocutionist gets into the habit of creating both the characters whom he is supposed to be addressing when not speaking directly to the audience and the scenes associated with the piece he has in hand...*

"Elocution", he added, *"is being studied in England today much more widely than it ever was before. The tendency is to regard it as an essential brand of study in all good schools, and whereas formerly the schoolmasters themselves used to teach what little was taught, now, finding that they have not the time, if even they have the knowledge, they consider it necessary to employ specialists....Alluding to the selection of poems for the platform, Mr Campbell observed that there was a great demand in the present day for the humorous and pathetic, and a corresponding lack of appreciation for the classic.*

"Of Australian pronunciation Mr Campbell expressed a not unnatural horror. At the same time he did not think the affliction incapable of cure, and said that during the course of some months spent in Tasmania in search of health after the fatigues of professional work during a severe English winter, he succeeded in effecting a marked improvement in the speech of a class of girls at the Ladies' School, Launceston."

The Melbourne Shakespeare Society, one of a number of such societies in Australia, most of which came and went, was founded in 1884 and still exists. The founding of this society brought together both University of Melbourne people and enthusiastic amateurs. As well as the reading of plays there were occasional entertainments for charity; the undertaking of critical studies of selected works; the publishing of relevant essays, and annual prize examinations relating to a set play. The membership of the society was large, some of the play readings were reported in the press and strong views were expressed in correspondence. On the lighter side Shakespeare's birthday on April 23rd was usually celebrated with some type of social function. Another group in existence in Melbourne for a time was the Roscians, a group founded by an Irish actor and playwright, Edmund Duggan, and others to provide for Shakesperean play readings.

The Alliance Francaise was founded in Melbourne in 1890 to help people become familiar with French language and culture. It still exists today and offers a wide range of activities. There had been a long tradition of leadership in France in the theatre arts of mime and movement. French was the language of diplomacy, study of French was considered important in Australia then and there was admiration for French culture and fashion.

It is well to remember that the percentage of the Melbourne population who would have had sufficient keenness to take part in cultural activities would have been comparatively small. Often there were people who belonged to one or more societies, so there was cross-linking. A number of the influential Melbournians who belonged to the various local clubs and societies were to become helpful contacts for FM Alexander in the 1890's, and in some cases became his pupils when he established himself in Melbourne as a vocal art teacher in 1896.

Lectures were another form of entertainment that could attract large crowds. Topics were diverse; educational, scientific, or cultural in nature, presentations varied. If the speaker was well-known, for example the British author Anthony Trollope, then Melbourne paid attention. Three thousand people attended his lecture in 1871 in the Town Hall on "Modern Fiction as a Rational Amusement'. As well as the main clubs of Melbourne, the suburbs had a wide variety of associations to cater for the peoples' tastes in mime, theatre, choirs, sport, recitation etc.

No reference to Melbourne however, would be complete without mention of the Melbourne Cup, a horse race begun in the year 1861, run on the first Tuesday of November and which even today brings the nation to a standstill while people wait to hear if their favourite has come in a winner. This race is the centrepiece of the Victorian racing calender; in the Centennial year of 1888 over 100,000 people were estimated to have attended Australia's premiere horse race. Horses had been an integral part of FM Alexander's life - he rode, his father was a blacksmith, no doubt FM Alexander developed a very knowledgable eye when it came to assessing the qualities of a horse, its gait, its potential. A hobby which FM pursued throughout his life was to have a bet on the races and coming to Melbourne would have allowed him to experience the excitement of race days, along with many other Melbournians, from all walks of life, who regarded racing as a most enjoyable pastime.

F. M. ALEXANDER IN MELBOURNE

After the first few months of exploring what Melbourne cultural life had to offer, FM did what most aspiring young artists have to do, took jobs to earn money, while continuing his artistic studies. In those days there was no drama college for a formal degree course. Study for a stage career could be approached in various ways. It was possible to take part in amateur theatricals to gain experience, then hope to make the transition to the professional stage. An experienced actor might be willing to offer coaching and then possibly employ this "apprentice" in small parts. There were a number of elocution teachers who offered training in all aspects of vocal art.

Because of his work experience at Waratah and the degree of competency that he had shown there, FM had no difficulty in securing employment in Melbourne. During his five years in this city (1889-1893) FM worked initially for a dairy produce auctioneering company then spent 18 months with a department store, George and George. This exclusive shop in Collins Street Melbourne is still in operation, now known simply as Georges. FM's health, which was not robust, gave him increasing problems, so on the advice of his doctor, Dr.Charles Bage, he moved to the sea-side town of Geelong, some 72 kilometres away. Here he was able to work for a local department store for six months, and then with improved health returned to Melbourne to obtain a position with a tea merchant company. These clerical and accounting jobs provided him with the means for existence and for his developing study of all aspects of drama.

One of FM's teachers was Mr F. W. Hill, the son of T. P. Hill, who had written a book, 'The Oratorical Trainer, A System of Voice Culture'. This book was referred to as a standard Australasian work on elocution, copies of which can still be seen in the State Library of Victoria. It was first printed in 1862 and went through many printings until the early 1900's. It was the text book recommended by the Teachers and Schools Registration Board who from 1907 had Government authority to register teachers at non-Government Schools. The category for teachers of special subjects included the teaching of Elocution. (See latter part of chapter 10.)

Thomas Padmore Hill (1820-1879) was born in Middlesex, England. His early career as a journalist took him to Mauritius and the Cape of Good Hope. In the early 1850's he came to Adelaide where he spent several years as journalist and lecturer. From 1858 until his death, Melbourne was his place of residence and his chief occupation was as a teacher of elocution, though he maintained some journalistic connections. T. P. Hill held the position of master of elocution at Scotch College, and also taught at Melbourne Church of England Grammar School, Wesley College, St Patrick's College and other schools.

An old Scotch Collegian writing his memories of staff in those times recalled, "*T. P. Hill was our instructor in elocution, and a splendid teacher he was, and a grand speaker, too. I can still fancy I hear him, as he stood before his class in the big English Room, giving his orders thus: 'Head erect, body slightly inclined forward, well supported on the lower limbs, chiefly resting on the right foot.'*" Mr Hill's main teaching work in his later years was for the State Government Education Department as a lecturer on elocution to State School teachers in Melbourne, Geelong and Ballarat.

The Oratorical Trainer, A System of Voice Culture by T. P. Hill, contains detailed instruction for speech, and many examples from the literature which could be used for performance. Hill states: "*a cultivated and well modulated voice always commands attention, and enlists the sympathies of an audience.*" Included in the Introduction are references to the importance of improving the elocution of the clergy and the need for better teaching of reading in schools. "*The study of a good delivery should commend itself to every educator of youth.*" The author concludes the Introduction by saying his aim is "*to make the study of the art of delivering written and spoken language easy, delightful, and instructive.*" In the 1890's when F.M.Alexander wrote his own articles on elocution, he quoted liberally from The Oratorical Trainer.

The main part of The Oratorical Trainer begins :

"*ELOCUTION is the art of delivering written and spoken language in a manner that shall vividly represent the conceptions of an author, or impress upon an audience the full force of a speaker's original effusions. The prime requisites of a good delivery are -*

I. A PROPER MANAGEMENT OF THE BREATH.

II. CLEAR AND DISTINCT ENUNCIATION.

III. CORRECT PRONUNCIATION.

IV. THE ABILITY TO EMPLOY THE UPWARD OR DOWNWARD SLIDES OF THE VOICE SO AS TO FASTEN THE MIND ON THE SENSE OF WHAT IS READ OR SPOKEN.

V. MODULATION OF THE VOICE, AND THE POWER OF SUBORDINATING WORDS TO IDEAS.

VI. *DISCRIMINATING EMPHASIS.*

VII. *JUDICIOUS PAUSATION.*

VIII. *A GOOD OROTUND TONE.*

IX. *GRACEFUL GESTURE.*

X. *EARNESTNESS.*

Then follows fourteen preliminary directions including,
" 2. *Inflate the lungs with air inhaled through the NOSTRILS.* (The process of inspiration and respiration must be perfectly effortless.)*
** There are two good reasons for this recommendation. First, because it greatly facilitates vocal exertion; and, secondly, because the nostrils, by means of their delicate and fibrous linings, purify and warm the air in its passage to the lungs. In a sanitary point of view, therefore, the practice is very important."*

The 1867 edition of The Oratorical Trainer contains a number of testimonials to the efficacy of Mr Hill's teaching and reviews of the book by a wide cross-section of the Colonial Press.
Mr. Alex Morrison, A. M., Principal, Scotch College; *"I have much pleasure in bearing testimony in favour of Mr. T. P. Hill, Professor of Elocution at the Scotch College. He has conducted large public classes in this institution for five years."*
Mr. W. J. Stephens, M.A. Oxon., Headmaster of the Sydney Grammar School; *"I have much pleasure in expressing the very high estimate which I have formed of your skill, zeal, and success as a teacher of elocution. In the short space of six weeks....the general improvement in voice and articulation has been very marked, while the speeches with which we are accustomed to close each quarter exhibited an extraordinary progress in declamation."*

"LECTURING TOUR IN TASMANIA

Mr. Hill's success has been universal. Wherever he has appeared he has been acknowledged a master of the Art of Elocution. - Launceston Chronicle.

Mr. T. P. Hill. - This gentleman made his last public appearance in Hobart Town on Monday evening. The room was densely crowded, a large number of persons being unable to find admission. Mr. Hill gave several recitations with great effect. As Mr. Hill is on the point of leaving the colony, we must put on record our high sense of the service he has rendered to the cause of education here, by directing attention to a branch of it that is by far too much neglected. His Excellency the Governor and Lady Young patronised the performance. - Hobart Town Mercury.

LECTURING TOUR IN NEW SOUTH WALES

Last evening, PROFESSOR HILL's farewell drawing-room entertainment took place in the hall of the Australian Library. The hall was crowded by the elite of our city, amongst whom were his Grace Archbishop Polding and several clergymen of different denominations. PROFESSOR HILL's reception by his audience, throughout his entertainment, was most enthusiastic. - Sydney Empire, June 26, 1863.

A compilation like the one in question (The Oratorical Trainer) *cannot fail to prove a great boon, not only to those who are desirous of improving themselves in the delightful art of reading aloud with correctness and taste, but also to those who have not the means of a ready access to a large collection of books, as they will find, ready to their hand, a choice collection of pieces remarkable for interest and beauty of language. A plain and easily-comprehended code of instructions for the student of the art of elocution is prefixed to the volume. - Lyttelton Times, (New Zealand) May 28, 1864."*

Thomas Padmore Hill married Cecilia Hamilton Aycliffe at Christ Church, St.Kilda in 1859. She had been born in 1839, aboard ship travelling out from England, surely a hazardous beginning. Their only son, Frederick Wyndham Hill, was born in Melbourne in 1862. When T. P. Hill died in 1879 there were newspaper obituaries, including one in the Herald, Saturday November 29th, 1879, extracts as follows:

"Mr. Hill was well known and appreciated by a large circle of personal friends in literary and dramatic circles; and his wide range of information, experience, and ready command of language, made him a brilliant conversationalist and debater......

Mr. Hill was also well known in newspaper circles, and was a frequent and valued contributor to the columns of THE HERALD, principally, however, on dramatic subjects. An ardent admirer of the drama, and an acute and thoughtful critic, his writings were laden with good scholarly criticism, devoid of conventionalism, and giving sign of careful consideration..... He was an enthusiast in his profession, and frequently contributed to these columns valuable papers on elocution, public reading, and speech culture."

Little is known about F. W. Hill, the voice teacher of F.M.Alexander, who did not have the same high profile as his father. It seems he did not teach elocution in schools but had his own private teaching studio in Melbourne. On November 13th, 1891, Table Talk notes: *"The Olympians give an entertainment in aid of the Gordon Institute and the Try Class of Melbourne at St. George's Hall, Bourke-street, on Wednesday, November 25. Mr. F.W.Hill, professor of elocution, is the club's managing director of the rehearsals."* F.M.Alexander apparently developed a strong connection with this group, see page 51 the May 19th 1893 review of a performance given by the Olympians. By the late 1890's F. W. Hill had developed a dual career. In 1897 his entry in the Sands and MacDougall Street Directory was as follows: " *HILL F. WYNDHAM, Professor of Elocution and shorthand writer and instructor. Chancery Lane, Melbourne and Toorak."*

In 1909 F. W. Hill ceased to list himself in the Directory as a teacher of elocution. This could have been for two reasons, the growing demand for his services as a shorthand writer, and the fact that elocution as a study was declining in popularity. (See the latter part of Chapter 10 re elocution and the Teachers and Schools Registration Board.)

When F.W.Hill died in 1936, the Argus newspaper of October 3rd, 1936, noted: " *Mr Frederick Wyndham Hill, of Millicent avenue, Toorak who died in a private hospital yesterday morning, was one of the most widely known professional shorthand writers in Melbourne. He was aged 75 years, and had been ill for some weeks. He was well known, not only at the Law Courts but also as the proprietor of a shorthand school in Chancery Lane, and as the official reporter for a number of racing clubs."*

When F. M. Alexander subsequently travelled in Tasmania and New Zealand, he was to refer in respectful terms to the elocutionary soundness of the work of both T.P.Hill and his son, F.W.Hill. But in the early 1890's FM was developing his dramatic skills in amateur performances. The Age (Melbourne daily) of November 26th, 1891 noted, " *Mr F. M. Alexander gave a tragic recital with great spirit."*

Drama and music competitions, whether in the form of an eisteddfod or similar event, have long offered the opportunity for artists to try their wings. In 1892 the Victorian Amateur Competitions Association ran a competition which was divided into musical, literary, dramatic and elocutionary sections. The Herald (a Melbourne daily) reported on September 14th, 1892 that section winners in the preliminary contests were: *"....Dialogue, Miss C. Malmgren and Mr F. M. Alexander ...The winning dialogue was chosen from Macbeth and was listened to with rapt and silent attention. Miss Malmgren and Mr Alexander received a most enthusiastic ovation at its conclusion, the applause continuing even as they walked down the hall after leaving the platform."*

In 1893 FM appeared as a recitalist with his own compostion and The Reformer noted on May 14th, 1893, *"An original recital "The Dream of Matthias the Burgomaster', contributed by F. M. Alexander, showed that gentleman to be possessed of great histrionic abilities, and he afterwards favoured with a pathetic recital, which was splendidly rendered, a recall being demanded for each item".* A year previously Table Talk (Melbourne Weekly) of May 13th 1892 noted: *"It would be against the canons of newspaper writing to start a reference to an unknown poet without quoting Gray's line, "Some mute, inglorious Milton," so now the quotation is made attention may be drawn to a poem, "published for the first time, by Mr. Fred. M. Alexander, of Newton House, Scott Street, St. Kilda." It is entitled "The Dream of Matthias the Burgomaster," and was written after witnessing Mr. Bentley as Matthias in The Bells. The piece is well adapted for recitation, and possesses considerable literary merit. The following verse is a fair sample of the poem: -*

He tried to sleep, but all in vain, his eyes were hot and red,
The vision was before him now, it hovered round his bed;
With trembling frame and haggard face he moved about the room,
For the human blood that he had shed now seemed to seal his doom."

"The Bells" was an adaptation by Leopold Lewis of a play by Erckmann-Schatrian, called Le Juif polonais - The Polish Jew. It was a melodramatic play about Matthias the Burgomaster and the character of Matthias was one of the British actor, Henry Irving's great parts. The plot, about a guilty murderer, is also the theme of Thomas Hood's poem, "the Dream of Eugene Aram", part of the recitalist's repertoire.

A copy of The Dream of Matthias the Burgomaster by Fred. M.Alexander is in the National Library, Canberra. This copy has handwritten on it, to "Jas.Smith", this would no doubt have been the James Smith whose life was summarised earlier. It is not a formal dedication, but it is most probable that FM would have known James Smith and sent him a copy of his poem. James Smith had always been a collector of books and other literature and kept an extensive library at his Melbourne home. When he died in 1910, the disposal of his books was advertised as follows, *"Important Auction Sale of a Valuable Library of Books. 5,000 volumes, including works on Fine Arts, Poetry, Biography, Historical, Political, English and French Fiction, Shakespeare, French Literature, Music and Drama, Travels, Science, Natural History, Australasian, and Rare and Valuable Australian Pamphlets".*

THEATRE ROYAL.

Lessees ...	THE AUSTRALIAN THEATRICAL MANAGEMENT CO., LIMITED
Managing Director	MR. GEORGE COPPIN
Acting Manager	MR. A. SULLIVAN
Treasurer	MR. R. F. KEATING

MONDAY, DECEMBER 7TH, 1891,

The Celebrated Tragedian, Mr.

WALTER BENTLEY

As "MATHIAS" (the Burgomaster) in "**The Bells**," for the First Time in the Colonies, and "JOCK HOWIESON" in "**Cramond Brig**."

EVERY EVENING AT EIGHT—The Powerful Melodrama,

THE BELLS

Or, The Murder of the Polish Jew.

Mathias	(The Burgomaster)	WALTER BENTLEY
Christian		Mr. JULIUS KNIGHT
Father Walter		MR. J. F. CATHCART
Dr. Zemmer		Mr. R. CRAWFORD
Sozel		Miss GWENDOLYN FLOYD
Judge		Mr. E. STEVENS
Clerk		Mr. A. HILL
Annette		Miss LAURA HANSEN
Hans		Mr. ALBERT BERNARD
Notary		Mr. E. MONEY
Tony		Mr. C. DRURY
Catherine		Miss EMILY STAFFORD
Mesmerist		Mr. A. MARSCHEL

Soldiers and Peasants.

To be followed by the Laughable Historical Scotch Farce,

CRAMOND BRIG

Or, THE KING AND THE MILLER.

Jock Howieson (The Miller)	WALTER BENTLEY
King James	Mr. A. CLIFTON ALDERSON
Tam Maxwell	Mr. A. HILL
Jabos	Mr. E. CRAWFORD
Neighbours Bairn	Mr. G. DRURY
Lindsay	Miss FLOYD
Birkie o' Birkie	Mr. E. STEVENS
Capt. of Archers	Mr. A. BERNARD
Beston	Mr. T. FOSTER
Grimes	Mr. E. MONEY
Tibbie	Miss E. STAFFORD
Marion	Miss LAURA HANSEN

Advertisement for "The Bells:, the Lorgnette, December, 1891

(Courtesy of La Trobe Collection, State Library of Victoria)

By 1893 FM had increased his repertoire and was finding opportunities for performance. The Sun of May 13th 1893 reported, *"The feature of the second part of the entertainment was the recitation of Mr F. M. Alexander, who gave a pathetic recital 'Caoch the Pipper', an original piece of considerable literary merit entitled 'The Dream of Matthias the Burgomaster' and afterwards appeared in the Cottage scene from `The Honeymoon'. A good voice, wide range of emotional expression, and much dramatic force, should with careful training, carry their possessor to eminence upon the stage".*

Soon after, a Shakespearean evening was organised by the Olympians at the Hibernian Hall and attended by a large number of friends. The Sun of May 19th, 1893, reported *"Extracts from some of Shakespeare's best pieces were well given. Mr F. M. Alexander was indefatigable in his efforts to make the affair successful, his dramatic power being well shown in the murder scene from Macbeth, and in the two scenes from Hamlet, in each of which he took the name part. ..The jealousy scene from Othello was well performed - Mr F. M. Alexander as the Moor, Mr Tullett as Iago, while Miss C. Milton and Miss A. Sylvester took the parts of Desdemona and Emilia".* Another report of the same evening by the Table Talk magazine of May 19th, 1893, noted, *"Mr F. M. Alexander appeared in 'Hamlet', 'Othello', and 'Macbeth', and was seen to great advantage, these powerful characters serving to show off his dramatic powers".*

The quality of professional recitation and the merit of those who were teachers of this art received some public attention. A long article, "Public Declamation" in Table Talk, May 12th, 1893 is worth quoting for the light it throws on attitudes to these topics, at the time when FM was reaching a standard that led him to embark on his own professional career.

Public Declamation

by Frances Tyrrell-Gill

"....the practice of recitation is fast becoming as notable a feature of our modern life as the practice of music. Not only at the celebrations of the different schools of elocution, but both in public and private, the University Conversazione, the Artists' evening, the drawing room At Home, recitation, equally with music, forms an indispensable part of the entertainment. ......

The pompous declaimer of the merest doggrel, although his want of cultivation may betray itself in every word he utters, speaks of himself as following the same profession as the man with natural endowments who has devoted years to the study of the rendering of either Shakespeare or Shelley. With so wide a divergence of qualifications and attainments, it is naturally a little difficult to know what people mean when they say they are devoted to either music or poetry. But it is much easier to see that when fashion sets the example, both music and poetry may, in a certain sense, become popularised, without any particular reference to the question of art. And fashion has just now decreed that music and recitation shall form a large part of her social entertainment. Everyone is supposed to either play or recite. And the plentitude of instructors, with or without qualifications, may be looked upon simply as the supply created by the demand. In some instances there will be the cultured artist, trained and prepared for his work, and who will seek for love of art to awaken a kindred love in his pupil; but who can doubt that in the majority of instances the teacher will look upon his work as mere means to an end; will aim himself at being popular; and instead of endeavouring to awaken this true feeling for art, will inflate his pupils with the idea of making the whole matter a successful show. In short, he regards it from the monetary point of view only. The large amount of showiness and flimsiness shown in the rendering of both music and poetry, not only declares the shallowness of the motive that prompts the performance, but the kind of influence that lies behind it.

Here we have the youth, either on the platform of his particular school or society, or at "The Evening," given by his admiring relatives and friends, delivering himself, with uncultivated voice, and much inappropriateness of gesture, of some moving tale of flood and field."

The writer continues this theme about quality of performance and in reference to performers with more experience asks, " *Is it possible that these people can have deluded themselves into believing that all this strenuousness of voice and manner, this excessiveness of gesticulation, all this artificiality of attitude and movement, could really be called the interpretation of poetry?*

As far as performance goes, this unsatisfactory state of affairs, at least with reference to poetry, arises, doubtless, in some degree on the part of uncultured people, from a confusion of terms. They desire, as they assert, to study elocution, but their thoughts are all the while set upon recitation, the delivery before an audience of a composition committed to memory. The manner of its delivery will speedily show its raison d'etre. It may be wholly a matter between the reciter and his teacher whether his gestures shall be utterly unrelated to the sentiments expressed, as though having been learned by rote like the words they were to be given off in rotation, hands uplifted here, outstretched or wrung, together there, or whether the words themselves shall be rendered with full sympathy of tone, and the gesture itself arise naturally and harmoniously in its place. Elocution, on the contrary, is the art of speaking. It may, en passant, be observed that the masters whose names have weight, both of this and the kindred art of singing, not only make voice-culture an important part of their system, but train their pupils upon the same method.

Thus, the one refers to an act, the other to an elaborate study; for though elocution may reach its finest effects in recitation, recitation frequently shows that it has nothing whatever to do with elocution. But as long as this non-intelligent acceptation of the two words, as though they were convertible, remains, so long will there be adventitious display in place of beauty of voice and true expressiveness of look and bearing.

We have indeed in our midst teachers of elocution, who have not only perfect command of the techniques, but take a lofty view of their work; and who, having culture at their command, aim not only at making their pupils breathe, speak, look and move in complete harmony with the thoughts and emotion to which they are giving utterance, but endeavour to awaken a true understanding of such thought and emotion. For that primal canon in the interpretation of art, which has been noticeably revived of late in the question of music, applies with equal force to poetry - that it all lies, not so much in the exactness of every note rendered, but in the truth of the phrasing. Were there but a truer public understanding of this matter there would be a revolution in the way in which both music and poetry are generally rendered."

Some of the sentiments expressed in the above article were to find echoes in two articles written by FM when he was in Tasmania (1894) and New Zealand (1895). Both articles are in Chapter 9. The Tasmanian "Elocution As An Accomplishment", is quoted in full and the New Zealand "Speech Culture and Natural Elocution" in part.

INTERLUDE

During these years of working at daytime jobs, studying to be a reciter, developing a repertoire and taking engagements as they came along, FM had been troubled on and off by voice and breathing problems, which at times interfered with his performance. He worried about accepting engagements, fearing he might break down and not be able to conclude an evening recitation. FM sought advice from voice specialists and doctors who were unable to give him more than temporary relief from his problems. It looked like the end of a promising stage career. So he embarked on a series of experiments regarding his use of voice.

Working patiently and with perseverance, he learned to observe, with increasing awareness for fine detail, just how he was putting himself under unnecessary strain, not only around the neck area but throughout his whole musculature, in order to recite. This time of experimentation brought great and unexpected rewards. Not only did FM solve his voice problems but the knowledge and understanding which he gained, a result of this personal research, enabled him to become a unique teacher. Initially FM was a vocal art teacher, but ultimately the principles that he discovered led him to teach pupils how to improve the 'Use of the Self' in any given activity.

The following summary of what has become known as The Alexander Technique is put here to give readers who have not had Alexander lessons, an outline of FM Alexander's work as it is known today.

Alexander's methods involve a pupil learning improved understanding and perception of the head/neck/back relationship and how to maintain this relationship (not hold a position) in a chosen activity, ranging from one lasting a few seconds (like changing from standing to sitting), to more intricate and complex activities such as those of music or sport. This new organisation of oneself involves the changing of habit patterns - sometimes habits which have been acquired over many years. So the thinking is the key to the Alexander work, learning to inhibit a habitual response to a stimulus and learning to choose a more appropriate way to respond.

FM developed his work over many years, beginning in Melbourne in the early 1890's. He left no detailed records of this development, but at least his (at times detailed), teaching and performance advertisements give some clues to his unfolding journey, with indications of those who influenced his work. To date there has been no biography of FM, and he only left a sketchy unpublished autobiography, written late in life, about his years to 1904. He lived until 1955 and there is much original research to be done.

The 1890's, FM's initial years of research are now one hundred years away. Records of work by his pupils and colleagues in Australia are probably gone, though it is surprising what can turn up. Old magazines and newspapers are reasonable sources for information. With the increasing attention world-wide being given to FM Alexander's work, there will probably be more interest in, and more conjecture about how and why he developed as he did. This could lead to the publishing of material about FM Alexander, the man, which would give a broader picture of his life and times. This would be a useful addition to the already substantial number of books about the Alexander Technique.

When FM first tried his wings as a professional reciter with his Tasmanian tour of 1894, he had not decided that the stage would be his only career. Throughout his working life in Australia, (he went to England in 1904), FM combined both a stage and vocal art teaching career. The teaching was the more sustained and ultimately became his life's purpose, but for the Australian years, FM's love of the theatre never went too far below the horizon.

In those times there were certainly some actors who would have had exaggerated mannerisms. Also some theatres were large, having space for 1,500 to 3,000 patrons. With no microphones, adequate voice projection would have been essential, and no doubt the manner in which this was done would have been injurious to the health of some. FM mostly did recitations, which were usually given in smaller halls, but if he imitated some aspects of the exaggerated styles he observed, this could have contributed to his problems of vocal strain and general stress. He was of slight build and supposedly not of strong constitution, therefore undue effort would have told on him much more readily than on those in more robust health.

In his book, 'The Use of the Self' (published in 1931), Chapter One, where he describes how he evolved his own methods, FM does not give detail of his study experiences in Melbourne. There is reference to his memory of a teacher, (and this is forty years after the event), a Mr.James Cathcart having told him *"take hold of the floor with your feet"*, because he was not pleased with the way FM was standing and walking. FM realised much later that he had responded to this instruction by gripping and tightening his feet and making extra tension there; this tension had then spread throughout his whole musculature.

FM was first in Melbourne from about 1888 to the end of 1893. During this time, apart from seeing a great deal of theatre (and there was much to choose from) FM would most likely have been to more than one voice or elocution teacher. There are no records of this, only conjecture. However, when FM returned to Tasmania for his acting tour of 1894, the name of a teacher he worked with in Melbourne does appear in a review of his performance. The manner in which it appears suggests that FM was using the name as evidence of study with a successful Melbourne teacher. The teacher's name is F.W. Hill, son of T.P. Hill, who had written the Oratorical Trainer, described as the standard Australasian work on elocution. When budding artists first turn professional it is quite usual to put in the name of their teacher, particularly if that person is well-known. One cannot infer that this named teacher contributed to FM's performance difficulties. Rather, as he published the teacher's name it is more likely that this teacher is one for whom he would have had respect.

FM was able to solve the voice problems which had beset him and which had threatened to thwart his stage ambitions. With improved voice resonance and fine breath control, his confidence returned, and he was able to think seriously regarding his stage career. What better place to test the professional waters than in his home colony, Tasmania?

ON TOUR - TASMANIA AND NEW ZEALAND

FM Alexander returned to the island colony for a series of recitations, starting on the North West coast, at his home town of Wynyard, then moving to Launceston and finally to Hobart, the capital. This occupied several months of 1894.

The Wellington Times, a North West coast newspaper, announced in February 1894 that there would be *"A Grand Performance in aid of the funds of the Wynyard Brass Band in the Wynyard Town Hall on Wednesday next. February 21st. Mr F. M. Alexander (who secured First prize at the recent competition held in Melbourne, when he appeared in the title role of Shakespeare's sublime tragedy 'Macbeth', and also holds splendid criticisms from the daily, evening, society and other newspapers in Victoria), has generously conceded to give some of his FINEST RECITALS. He will be assisted by several talented ladies and gentlemen"*. Of the twenty items on the programme, FM contributed nine; they included his own poem, The Dream of Matthias the Burgomaster, excerpts from plays and humorous, tragic, sensational and pathetic poems. A full list of the poems Alexander recited as taken from newspaper advertisements and critiques, is at the end of the book. There was another Alexander who took part in the program that night. FM's sister Amy sang one song.

In Launceston local artists combined with FM for an evening of entertainment on May 10th, 1894. The Daily Telegraph reported,.... *"The 'Progress of Madness' was then recited by Mr F. M. Alexander, an elocutionist new to Launceston audiences, and who was the centre of attraction during the evening. Mr. Alexander possesses a good voice, as well as dramatic talent of no mean order, and gave a realistic conception of the piece. The strain on the elocutionist must have been considerable, for it is certainly no easy task to give eight recitations in one night. For a pathetic recitation, entitled 'Keeping His Word', Mr Alexander was deservedly recalled, while his versatility was displayed to advantage in the humorous recitations 'After Marriage' and the 'Country Squire'. The elocutionist also gave 'Parrhasius'; Marc Antony's famous speech over the dead body of Caesar; a very tragic composition of his own , which savours somewhat of 'Eugene Aram' and is entitled 'The Dream of Matthias, the Burgomaster', and 'The Midnight Charge' ..It was announced that Mr F. M. Alexander - to whom a very high compliment was paid - intended to remain in Launceston as a teacher of elocution. The entertainment was brought to a close with the National*

Anthem". This recital was given at the Mechanics Institute, Launceston and was followed by another one at nearby Lefroy on Saturday May 19th, 1894.

In his Launceston and Lefroy programmes FM was assisted by various supporting artists, including Mr and Mrs A. H. Bowden, who were both prominent musicians. Alfred H. Bowden was descended from an early Tasmanian family, he studied music in Hobart under Mr A.J.Dentith, who himself had studied music in Germany and England. Alfred Bowden then lived and worked in Melbourne for a time, took up music as his profession and for many years commanded respect for his musical activities in Tasmania, chiefly in Launceston. He was a violinist and choral and orchestral conductor. Mr Bowden's wife, the daughter of his Hobart music teacher, was herself a talented pianist and highly successful music teacher.

The announcement in early May that FM intended to stay a while in Launceston as a teacher of elocution was repeated at the end of May. 'The Tasmanian' on May 26th noted, *"Mr F. M. Alexander, the clever young elocutionist, has determined to sojourn in Launceston for a time and give instruction in voice culture"*. In early June there was an announcement that FM would give one of his elocutionary entertainments in Hobart. This took place on June 29th at the Hobart Town Hall. It is interesting to note that two of the other performers were Mr.and Mrs R.Young. Both were associated with FM in performance and as teaching colleagues in subsequent years. The critique for this Hobart Town Hall performance from The Mercury of June 30th, 1894 included the following:

"Mr. Alexander well established himself in public favour, judging from the enthusiastic applause accorded him. He proved his elocutionary ability to be of a high order, and showed himself capable of dealing with any subject - grave or gay, tragic or comic.......

Mr Alexander was ably assisted by Mrs. R. Young in the quarrel scene from the School for Scandal, and Miss E. Miller in a selection from Tobin's comedy, The Honeymoon. Both ladies exhibited considerable dramatic ability, and were accorded flattering approval.....

Mr. R. Young revived his merry acquaintanceship with the Hobart public in Grossmith's sketch, "The silver wedding," and his return was greeted with manifest approval. He filled the audience with unmeasured merriment throughout his performance."

The success of his Hobart visit decided FM to stay in that city and teach voice culture. His Melbourne training and drama experience combined with his developing skill in analysing and improving his performance ensured a degree of confidence, illustrated by an article he wrote for the Hobart Mercury, July 9th, 1894.

ELOCUTION AS AN ACCOMPLISHMENT.

(By F. M. ALEXANDER)

"I would rather be called a "natural elocutionist," because I am afraid the word elocutionist is so much associated with a person possessing an artificial voice, unnatural style, unnatural inflection, and that most dreaded and unpardonable fault which is commonly known as staginess. This idea is so firmly rooted amongst theatrical managers that the mere mention of the word "elocution" by a young person seeking an engagement is sufficient to cause the application to be promptly declined.

"As a matter of fact the class of voice users to which I refer should not be termed "elocutionists." However, the term is so commonly misapplied that I make a distinction by referring to the matter as the art of natural elocution. C. T. Hartley, professor of elocution, London, Oxford, and Cambridge, has taken this view, and has published a little work called "Natural Elocution," which all reciters and speakers should carefully "read, mark, learn, and inwardly digest." Few people are born elocutionists, in the proper sense of the word, and thus so many fall into grievous errors. I say to all, "Hold the mirror up to Nature," and learn to feel, and in these few words we have the great secret of a speaker's success. The finest effects are produced by intensity, and not by loudness. This is a great error, into which so many fall. To quote Hartley, "The power of condensed energy in repose, with an accompanying clearness of enunciation which renders the suppressed whisper as impressive as the loudest explosion of agony, is a mastery of the art which none but the most highly gifted and persevering can attain." The tragic recital "Parhassius," included in my repertoire, calls into play the art to which Hartley refers, and without such treatment all the great effects of the composition could not be produced.

"My system of voice culture may be referred to under two headings; Voice building (an expression used by my teacher), and voice production, used together when training a weak voice, but with one of full power the voice production is all that is required. A comparatively weak voice can by these systems be built up to the ordinary power, and even the weakest can be materially strengthened. It so frequently happens that voices lack power on account of imperfect production, and to exercise such a voice without the assistance of an accomplished teacher, would be productive of the very worst results.

"The clergy are great sufferers from this cause, and Lennox Browne and Emil Behnke, when referring to the matter of "Clergyman's sore throat," bear

out this statement, and quoted numerous cases. Many have frequently to abandon their calling for months together, while others are always suffering with the throat. A course of careful training would remedy this, and their speaking would become a work of pleasure instead of a painful labour, and what a great blessing would be conferred upon their hearers. Dr. Johnson gave the following advise to a young clergyman : - "Delivery is more potential than eloquent matter," and the celebrated preacher, the Rev. John Wesley, said, " Take care of anything awkward or affected in your gesture, phrase, or pronunciation." The remarks just quoted are as applicable to barristers as to the clergy, and voice training is one of the first studies to which they should turn their attention; a good voice being an absolute necessity to enable them to thoroughly and effectively carry out their respective callings. Lord Chesterfield says, "I have frequently known a man's fortune decided for ever by his first address. You will make it your business, your study, and your pleasure, to speak well if you think right." This is indeed golden advice.

"How frequently we listen to members of the professions mentioned dealing with a good subject in well chosen words, but as they lack a voice which commands attention, little impression is made, and the listeners become so wearied with the delivery, that they feel disgusted with the subject, and the speaker's words fall upon the ear 'like sounding brass and a tinkling cymbal.'

"Stuttering and stammering are terms as to which there is much confusion of ideas, and are generally considered to be one and the same thing, which is quite a mistake. To go into details on this matter would take some hours, but broadly speaking, stammering is "frequently due to defective physical formation," and stuttering to "spasmodic muscular contractions." A thorough master of voice culture can do much to remedy such defects, and of late years many cures have been effected. Curran, one of Ireland's finest orators, was at one time called "little stuttering Jack Curran," but by assiduously following a course of training he overcame this great failing.

"Unfortunately, voice training is much neglected, for even outside of the benefits mentioned the study of elocution necessitates the student becoming familiar with the very best literature, which must have an elevating and refining effect upon those who take up its study. Any person who uses his influence in endeavouring to arouse interest in this study is doing a truly great work, and if successful will command the sincere thanks of all concerned. I am forced to admit that I am interested from a financial standpoint, as one must live (to use an every day expression), but I am deeply interested in these arts from an educational point of view, and have always been considered a great enthusiast, and trust that the business side of my life will not crush that enthusiasm."

This article is the first known public statement by FM about his ideas on Elocution. He published a second, more detailed article in Auckland in July, 1895.

Both articles show influences as follows:

1. C.T.Hartley, professor of elocution, London, Oxford and Cambridge, from whose book, "Natural Elocution" FM quotes.

2. Lennox Browne and Emil Behnke.
Lennox Browne was an eminent surgeon in London in the latter part of the 1800's. His positions included; senior surgeon to the Central Throat and Ear Hospital and surgeon and aural surgeon to the Royal Society of Musicians. Emil Behnke was a lecturer on voice physiology and teacher of voice production.

Both men had written books in their own right, and they combined to produce " Voice, Song and Speech" which was first published in 1883, subsequently being reprinted many times, with wide circulation. The detailed section on breathing includes the following:

"It may be added that in lung gymnastics, as well as while using the voice, the process of breathing must be carried on in perfect silence. This applies more particularly to inspiration, which is frequently accompanied by more or less noise. ......"

"Mouth-breathing is a pernicious and dangerous practice which frequently leads to diseases of the respiratory and of the vocal organs, and which ought to be discarded as much as possible."

Pages 228-230 of this book contain a good summary about the difficulties of stammering and stuttering, information on which FM based his own observations.

3. T.P.Hill, author of The Oratorical Trainer. In the introduction to his book, T.P.Hill makes considerable mention of the need for the clergy to develop proficiency in voice use. Likewise FM, in both his articles, refers to this matter and even goes so far as to include, in the New Zealand article, a quotation on this topic by Rev. Hugh McNeile, D.D. from Hill's book. Also in the New Zealand article the quotations from Lord Brougham and The Times are from the Introduction to Hill's book. The last part of the New Zealand article quotes from T.P.Hill. The genius of FM lay in his ability to absorb information from various quarters, to experiment and analyse in the best

traditions of scientific investigation, and to build the results of his research into an overall view of the psycho - physical functioning of the human being. In 1894 FM was at the beginning of his lifelong research and teaching career.

Extracts from the Auckland Star, July 20th, 1895 article, Speech Culture and Natural Elocution by F.M.Alexander.

"Unfortunately, these important arts are very sadly neglected in the colonies, especially outside of the large Australian cities. This neglect is due in a great measure to the fact that an erroneous idea prevails that good delivery and the proper use of the speaking voice is the common gift of Nature, and not the product of art. ......

"Cultivated speaking voices are as rare as the oasis in the desert. The improvement that can be made by proper training is simply wonderful, and the most moderate voices can be extended in range, strengthened in power and rendered flexible to a remarkable degree. To acquire a good delivery should be the ambition of all, because, as Lord Brougham observes, `It enables a man to do at all times what nature only teaches on occasion.' True ease in reading and speaking as in writing,

' — comes from art, not chance.
As those move easiest who have learned to
dance
'Tis not enough no harshness give offence,
The sound must be the echo of the sense.'

"Nature may endow a person with splendid vocal organs but they cannot possibly be used to anything like proper advantage until thoroughly trained. Some years ago a series of excellent articles on the subject of speech culture appeared in the `Times,' the following being an extract: -

'From the time a gentleman's son goes to school, to the happy moment when he sees his name, perhaps on the list of wranglers on the class list, he has most probably, never recited English poetry or prose, never even read aloud, much less has he ever made an oral statement of fact to a greater length than a short sentence to a short question. Up to the age of three and twenty, it is a matter yet to be ascertained whether the intended clergyman can read a verse in the Bible as it ought to be read, whether the intended barrister can make a legal statement without giving disgust, or persuade without making himself ridiculous. He may at that age be able to do many things seldom required. He may be deep in Greek and Roman antiquities, and able to construe, and even to construe any chorus; he may write Latin and Greek verses in a dozen metres. He may be a good mathematician, and even compose a tolerable essay. He may have these and other accomplishments which may

never be called into practice in a whole life, except in the production of written sermons, or in some correspondence of unusual gravity. What, however, every man must do, in one way or another, what is the common gift of all classes and all professions, all ages from infancy; what is the first and foremost difference between man and brute, between one man and another, is left to chance, without any assistance whatever from schools or universities. The first education that the country can give offers no security whatever that a man shall not offend and disgust when he should please and inform. Enter church after church, in the metropolis or elsewhere, and you will hear the prayers read by a machine and the sermon preached by a drone. This ought not to be, but it is so, and will remain so as long as the art of speaking is neglected in all its stages and applications, and nothing is cared for but head work and pen work, as applied to ancient languages and pure mathematics.'

"From the foregoing we find one of the foremost journals in the world giving great attention to this matter of speech culture, and doing a truly noble work in endeavouring to arouse interest in this all-important art. ....

"Dr. Johnson gave the following advice to young clergymen: — `Delivery is more potential than eloquent matter;' and the Rev. Hugh McNeile, D.D., wrote: `It would be difficult to estimate the advantage that might, under the Divine blessing, be derived from elocution classes in our universities, and if candidates for holy orders were thereby delayed a year, there would be more than compensation for the delay in the increased competency for the work.' We might cite a multitude of similar opinions from reverend gentlemen, but want of space prevents it. The remarks just quoted are as applicable to barristers as to clergymen, and voice training is one of the first studies to which they should turn their attention, a well cultivated voice being an absolute necessity to enable them to thoroughly and effectively carry out their respective callings. ......

"That great and highly esteemed authority, the late T. P. Hill (author of the well known `Oratorical Trainer,' now in its 12th edition) says that three of the great reasons that speech culture commends itself to public favour, are:-

'Because a well-cultivated and well-modulated voice always commands attention, and enlists the sympathies of an audience.'

'Because it places in the hands of one man the power of spreading the refining influences of literature amongst thousands who might be otherwise unconscious of them.'

'Because it begets a love for reading, which if formed in early life, will, by mere force of habit, last through life.'

And thus by the present neglect of speech culture we lose the great blessings that it would otherwise confer upon us by its refining influence, and the immense good which would result by its power in encouraging the love of reading in a great degree. We can each picture for ourselves the effect of such loss upon the whole community from this point of view."

The New Zealand Tour

After the success of his recitations in Tasmania, FM travelled to New Zealand; this country was very much part of a touring circuit followed by both overseas and local artists. Shipping was frequent between Melbourne, Hobart, Sydney and New Zealand ports. FM had a friend in Christchurch, New Zealand who assured him that a recital tour in New Zealand would have a good chance of success, so going there was a natural progression.

FM began his New Zealand tour in the city of Christchurch. As with the Tasmanian sojourn, FM gave recitations and taught. An advertisement in the Lyttelton Times, Christchurch for March 14th, 1895, stated, *"Natural Elocution, voice culture and dramatic training. Mr F. M. Alexander will receive pupils for the study of the above arts, and may be interviewed at his studio, Luck's Buildings, top floor Colombo Street, where original testimonials may be seen. Mornings 11 till 1; afternoons 4 till 6; evenings 8 till 10. Members invited to Shakespearean and Elocution classes. Terms - private, three pounds three shillings to five pounds five shillings per quarter; class, one pound ten shillings per quarter".*

On March 20th, 1895, a similar advertisement appeared but with some elaboration, *"where original testimonials may be seen from scholastic institutions, private pupils and the press...Elocution and Shakespearean classes now forming. Mr Alexander does NOT teach Elocution but Natural Elocution, the system adopted - by C. S. Hartley, professor of Natural Elocution, London, Cambridge and Oxford".*

The Lyttelton Times reported on April 6th that a recital by FM *"on Tuesday last was received with wild enthusiasm, Mr Alexander being recalled FIVE times during the evening. The press have been most eulogistic in their comments on the realistic impersonations of the varied characters assumed by Mr Alexander, and upon all that pertains to his elocutionary power as a MASTER".* FM gave further recitals and taught, then went to Wellington where again he had success as a reciter.

It was a general custom with performance advertisement, to be lavish and fulsome with descriptive phrases, perhaps more so than today. Certainly FM's advertisements show no lack of a complimentary turn of phrase. In

Wellington, the New Zealand Times, announced on April 30th, 1895, an FM recitation as follows, *"Dramatic, Artistic, Realistic, Humorous, Mr F. M. Alexander the versatile reciter and first prize winner in 'Macbeth' will appear at Thomas Hall, Thursday May 2nd and Monday May 6th. The press and public of Australia unanimously proclaim Mr. Alexander the most versatile reciter in the colonies. He appeared in Christchurch recently and was recalled five times during the evening, and the press unanimously pronounce him a THOROUGH MASTER. Amongst the gems to be given will be, 'The Dream of Eugene Aram', The Death of Poor Jo, Mark Antony's Oration, Kissing Cup's Race, and three humorous numbers. Fuller particulars to follow"*.

The critiques for his Wellington performances were equally praiseworthy. After Wellington FM had a brief visit to Napier, then paid a longer visit to Auckland, where he had many worthwhile opportunities to develop both his acting and teaching careers. News of FM's impending arrival in Auckland preceded him. The New Zealand Herald, May 18th, 1895:

"A Napier correspondent wires: "The Alexander-Blaney-Fisher Company will soon be with you. Mr Alexander is far and away the best elocutionist who has ever visited New Zealand and has a happy choice of pieces. He is a perfect host in himself. .... The company is a really first class one and the entertainment thoroughly refined and high class."

The following extracts from The New Zealand Herald outline the high points of FM's six month stay in Auckland.

June 6th, 1895 : "CITY HALL Monday next, June 10
Mr John Birch's Fifth Popular concert and dramatic performance. First production of a new one act play by John Birch entitled "Paul Daroon". The cast to include Madame Goldenstedt, Miss Matie Youlin, Mr. John Birch and Mr.F.M. ALEXANDER (of the Alexander-Blaney-Fisher Combination) who will create the title part."

June 10th, 1895 : "CITY HALL Tonight! Tonight! Tonight!
"Paul Daroon!" a new one-act play by John Birch. A Grand Concert! Eight first appearances. Full programme in Saturday's papers. Mr. F.M. Alexander (of the Alexander-Blaney-Fisher Combination) as "Paul Daroon". .... All who have heard Mr. F.M. Alexander recite during the short time he has been here, have beyond all doubt booked seats for tonight. Those who have not heard him have a treat in store."

June 11th, 1895 : "MR. JOHN BIRCH'S CONCERT ......
The play last night was well received. Mr. F.M. Alexander played admirably in the title role. Upon him much of the success of the piece depended."

As well as taking the leading role in this play FM was preparing for his first solo recital.

June 11th, 1895 : "CITY HALL
New and Novel entertainment, Thursday June 13th
MR. F.M. ALEXANDER
Pronounced by the southern press to be the most versatile actor-reciter and entertainer who has visited New Zealand in his Humorous, Pathetic and Sensational sketches from life."

June 14th, 1895 : "A NEW AND NOVEL ENTERTAINMENT
Last night there was a good attendance at the City Hall, when an excellent entertainment was given by Mr.F.M.Alexander and a well selected company engaged in support. Mr.Alexander, who is undoubtedly an able actor and reciter, first gave the stirring recitation "Kissing Cup's Race", for which he was compelled to reappear. He next gave from "The quarrel scene" in "The School for Scandal" an excellent interpretation of the character of Sir Peter Teazle, Madame Goldenstedt playing Lady Teazle admirably. Mr. Alexander's sketch from "The Tale of Two Cities" was an artistic effort as was also "Marc Antony's Oration."

On June 22nd there was a report of a concert with two singers, Miss Fisher and Miss Blaney, and Mr.F.M.Alexander. His critiques included :
June 22nd, 1895 : "Mr.F.M.Alexander first recited "The Amateur Rider" and was recalled. He then gave "The Dream of Eugene Aram" with artistic effect. With a voice under perfect control, with enunciation clear and distinct, and with fine dramatic force, he worked feeling up to keenest tension. The effect was a distinct success. Mr. Alexander also gave with pathos "our folks" in response to an encore, "the billiard-marker's story" which was one of his best."

Another talented lady, Miss Jessie Glover, engaged FM to play Romeo to her Juliet in scenes from that Shakespearean play for her performance on June 26th at the Opera House.

July 13th, 1895 : "AUCKLAND LITERARY SOCIETIES' UNION
Wednesday next, July 17th at 7.30 p.m. at Y.M.C.A. lecture hall CONVERSAZIONE ....
Grand Musical and Elocutionary entertainment in which the undermentioned will take part: Miss C.Lorrigan and Miss Brown, Mr F M Alexander, (The

talented elocutionist), Mr Apirana T Ngata, M.A. (The gifted Maori reciter), Mr R H A Potter and others."

During his Tasmanian and New Zealand visits FM was continuing to 'work on himself', that is, to make more and more detailed observations of the USE of himself in activity. Breathing and voice difficulties still bothered him but as he continued his observations about the relationship of the head/neck/back and how alteration of this relationship affected his performance - in any given activity, he gained new understanding of the whole psycho-physical mechanism. As well as observing his own USE, FM studied the manner and use of others. While in New Zealand he had the opportunity to observe the Maoris and later referred in his writing to their splendid example *of natural endowment from a breathing point of view.*

As lecture tours were part of the entertainment scene at the time, the public had the opportunity to hear talks on diverse topics. In 1895 in Auckland lectures were given by high profile visitors, including the actor, Walter Bentley, Professor Loisette, a memory expert, and Frederic Villiers, a war correspondent.

June 4th, 1895 : " OPERA HOUSE, Friday June 7th
The Passion Play
Positively one night only. Illustrated by beautiful pictures. Exhibited and lectured on by Walter Bentley. This marvellous exhibition of The Life and Death of Jesus Christ has been viewed by crowded audiences in all the Southern cities, who have been highly delighted."

In July Professor Loisette made a strong impression on the locals in Auckland. The New Zealand Herald again:

July 23rd, 1895: " THE WORLD FAMED MEMORY EDUCATOR
Prof A Loisette of London and New York will give his introductory lecture on memory at
City Hall July 30th at 8 p.m. Course of three instruction lectures to follow. Success guaranteed. Mind-wandering cured."

July 24th, 1895: " PROF A LOISETTE of London and New York
Who is admitted to be the greatest living memory psychologist will give his introductory lecture on memory City Hall July 30th 8 p.m."

July 27th, 1895: " HOW TO NEVER FORGET
...... " by my system", said Prof Loisette to a HERALD representative yesterday, "I abolish mind wandering absolutely so that a person can give his mind to a subject and concentrate himself mentally upon it. The assimilative

faculties are enabled to take everything into the brain instead of through the eye and ear principally. Nature never intended anyone to have a bad memory. The fault is that people have been trained to remember by simply repeating. I teach so that people can never forget." To do this means a revolution in the application of mental science, if not in mental science itself, and Prof Loisette is armed with a host of most eulogistic testimonials from the deepest and cleverest thinkers in the world of science, jurisprudence and letters, men whose names are world-renowned, and who have all of them averred that the results obtained from following the course have been marvellous."

July 30th, 1895: " CITY HALL this evening at 8 p.m.
under the distinguished patronage of His Excellency the Governor, the Right Honourable the Earl of Glasgow, and under the patronage of and in the presence of His Worship the Mayor J J Holland esq.
Prof A Loisette's wonderous lecture on Assimilative Memory. An opportunity you must not lose on any account."

August 1st, 1895: " Prof Loisette, the memory psychologist, gave yesterday evening at Sowerby's Hall the first of his series of instruction lectures on "assimilative memory". Over a hundred joined the class and extra seating accommodation to that provided had to be sought."

After great success in New Zealand Professor Loisette left Auckland on August 7th, 1895 for Sydney. Not only had the Professor given much whilst in Auckland, he had also received — from F. M. Alexander, according to the following eulogy which appeared in the New Zealand Herald on
August 10th, 1895:

" A MAGNIFICENT EULOGY FROM PROFESSOR LOISETTE

Auckland, August 6, 1895

This is to say that I find myself under many obligations to
Mr F M Alexander, the Natural Elocutionist. I read his article which appeared in the Auckland Star (partially quoted earlier in this chapter) and soon applied to him. I had increased in weight some fifty pounds during the past few years, and found as a consequence I would get out of breath in public speaking. I had tried the remedies of two distinguished elocutionists elsewhere, but with no benefit. In three lessons Mr Alexander set me right. As a test I will add that when I went on to the stage at the City Hall, July 30th, I really feared I could not get through with my address. I was so ill and fatigued with giving private lectures; but, thanks to the exercises prescribed by Mr Alexander, I encountered no difficulty, and in fact I found at the close of my remarks I was less exhausted than I had ever before been in my life.

Having heard Mr Alexander recite several selections, I am satisfied that all who wish to acquire the noble art of attractive and effective reading and speaking cannot do better than to place themselves under Mr Alexander's instructions.

I feel confident that if Mr Alexander were in London or New York, he would soon be recognised as a first-rate artist in his profession, and that he would soon command the highest terms paid to voice builders and genuine trainers for public reading and speaking.
(Signed) A. LOISETTE.

Mr Alexander wishes to announce that he has promised to meet the Professor in New York in April next, when he will make public appearances in that city, and as he will only be here for a short time, intending students should begin immediately.

Correct Breathing for Speakers and Singers taught in from three to six lessons. Fee. One pound, one shilling.

Natural Elocution. Voice Production, etc.

Stuttering (the cure of) a speciality. ....

Shakespearean and Elocution Classes meet each week. Members invited. Terms. One pound, ten shillings per quarter.

Further particulars may be obtained at the
STUDIO ROOM 314
Victoria Arcade."

The final reference to visiting lecturers pertains to the war correspondent, Mr Frederic Villiers.

August 17th, 1895: "Although the story of the Chino-Japanese war, of which Mr Villiers was an eye witness from the commencement of the hostilities until the taking of Port Arthur, will form perhaps the most attractive feature of the three lectures which he will give in the Opera House next week, the chief events, as well as many amusing incidents, of the eight previous campaigns in which he represented the London Graphic will be described. The subjects of the three lectures are announced in the present issue, and all of them will be illustrated by limelight reproductions of Mr Villiers sketches and photographs, of which those of the Port Arthur massacre are the only snapshots that were taken."

August 19th,1895: " Mr Villier's name and fame has travelled before him. Seldom has any lecturer attracted such enormous and delighted audiences throughout Australia and his visit to New Zealand has proved a continuation of his Australian success. .... A fact hitherto unprecedented is that we have the privilege of hearing news and particulars of the late struggle between the

Japanese and the Chinese fresh from the lips of an eye witness even before related in the Old Country."

August 23rd, 1895: "Another large and enthusiastic audience greeted Mr Frederic Villiers, the eminent war correspondent at the Opera House last evening when he delivered his second lecture in Auckland entitled, "Battles,Bivouacs and Banquets". Those who heard Mr Villiers in his opening lecture on Wednesday evening were loud in their praise of him, and a second acquaintance with so distinguished a personage considerably enhanced this opinion."

A month later a second eulogy to FM's work was published.

September 24th, 1895: " A SECOND EULOGY. —Mr Frederic Villiers, the great War Correspondent, writes:- " Northern Club, Auckland, September 16,1895. Dear Mr Alexander :
Thanks for your suggestions re Voice Production. I can now talk for nearly two hours with MUCH MORE COMFORT. Thanks also for the charming morning I spent with you and your art. I have never met anyone WITH SO VERSATILE A TALENT AS A RECITER. I shall follow your career round the world as a public entertainer with the keenest interest. Trusting to meet you in either New York or London. (Sd.) FREDERIC VILLIERS. " —
MR F M ALEXANDER wishes to announce that he leaves Auckland in December next, when he will appear in Australia prior to leaving for America and London. This just allows time for a single course of instruction. Full particulars at Studio, Room 314, Victoria Arcade."

FM's stay in Auckland drew to a close. The time came to prepare for his own farewell recital in that city.
November 16th, 1895: " UNDER THE PATRONAGE OF HIS WORSHIP THE MAYOR City Hall Wednesday next, complimentary farewell tendered by his students to MR F M Alexander, Natural Elocutionist, and the most versatile actor-reciter in Australasia."

November 19th, 1895: " The pupils and friends of Mr F M Alexander tender him tomorrow evening a complimentary benefit in the City Hall and a splendid testimonial will be presented as well. His abilities as an elocutionist and teacher of elocution have been thoroughly appreciated, as is evidenced by his time being wholly occupied in teaching pupils. As an elocutionist and versatile actor and reciter, he has shown his artistic capabilities, and there is little doubt in the wider sphere of labour to which he is going he will earn high distinction."

The programme for the Farwell Recital was:

PROGRAMME - PART I

1. Song. 'Anchored' (with pictorial illustrations)
MR HOWARD CHAMBERS
2. Piano Solo. 'Marche de Rakoczy'...Liszt
MRS ERNEST H. QUERRE
3. Recital. 'Kissing Cup's Race' or 'The Amateur Rider'
MR F. M. ALEXANDER
4. Song. 'Good-bye' (by request)... Tosti
MISS COLETTA LORRIGAN
5. Violin solo (selected)
HERR ZIMMERMAN
6. Song. (selected)
MISS LIZZIE WARREN
7. Recital. 'Jugurtha's Prison thoughts' or 'Parrhasius'
MR F. M. ALEXANDER

Presentation of Testimonial
Interval of five minutes

PART II

1. Recital. 'The Death of Poor Jo'
MR WALTER MOORE
(Mr Alexander's pupil, secured first place in recent competition)
2. Piano solo. 'Husarenritt'...Spindler
MRS ERNEST H QUEREE
3. Recital. 'How Bill Adams won the Battle of Waterloo'
(pictorially illustrated with slides never shown in Auckland)
MR F. M. ALEXANDER
4. Song. (selected) with pictorial illustrations
MISS COLETTA LORRIGAN
5. Song. 'The Wolf'...Shield
MR HOWARD CHAMBERS
6. Violin solo. (selected)
HERR ZIMMERMAN

Accompanist - MISS AMY BATES

To commence at 8pm sharp. Doors open at 7.30. Carriages at 10.

November 21st, 1895: " FAREWELL TO MR ALEXANDER
In the City Hall last evening, a very successful concert, tendered to Mr F M Alexander, the well-known elocutionist, as a farewell by his pupils, was held. The large audience bore ample testimony to his popularity and the admiration of the public for his talent. At the interval His Worship the Mayor, Mr J J Holland, on behalf of Mr Alexander's pupils, presented him with a handsome illuminated address, and in a short speech passed a high eulogy on the recipient. Mr Alexander heartily thanked the givers. ....
Mr Alexander was received with applause on each appearance, and his pieces were doubly encored. The versatility of his talent was well brought out in "Parrhasius" and "The Amateur Rider". The former is full of fine sentiment and passion, and deals with the thoughts of an artist; while the latter is the story of the stable. Yet he dealt with these two very opposite subjects in a most masterly manner, and held his audience spell-bound. He also recited "Kissing Cup's Race", "After Marriage" and "How Bill Adams Won the Battle of Waterloo".

After this highly successful New Zealand tour FM took ship to Sydney and then went by train to Melbourne which was to remain his base for the next four years.

TEACHING AND RECITING

Thus far FM Alexander had achieved success as a reciter and a teacher, but dual careers are difficult to maintain. FM made a decision to devote his energies to furthering his teaching career, but he did not neglect the stage for long.

He rented a teaching room in the Australian Building, 49 Elizabeth Street. This building was a landmark in Melbourne. At the time it was one of the tallest buildings in the Southern Hemisphere, being twelve storeys high and serviced by the new technology of hydraulic lifts. The building of this skyscraper in the late 1880's, at the height of the boom years, had been a source of public wonder and admiration. However, with the financial crash of the early 1890's office space was hard to let and many buildings, including the Australian Building, remained untenanted.

Other reasons for high buildings remaining empty, particularly those above two storeys, were that some customers were disinclined to trust the new fangled lifts, which were prone to break down, and at the time fire brigades only had equipment that could cope with two storeys in the event of fire, so special precautions had to be taken. Customers gradually were willing to travel higher and fire fighting equipment advanced. So when, in 1897, FM rented a studio on the seventh floor of the Australian Building there were several other tenants scattered through the higher floors. FM listed himself as a vocal art teacher.

FM's teaching practice developed reasonably but he felt that in order to become more widely known he needed to give recitals. This brought more pupils, the practice flourished and so too did FM's recitation work, to the point where he undertook recital engagements not only in Melbourne, but elsewhere.

The Age (a Melbourne daily newspaper) of May 11th, 1898, carried a large advertisement headed:

'ATHENAEUM HALL TONIGHT
First Appearance in Melbourne of
F. M. ALEXANDER F. M. ALEXANDER F. M. ALEXANDER
The VERSATILE ACTOR-RECITER, ENTERTAINER and NATURAL ELOCUTIONIST in an ENTIRELY NEW and NOVEL ENTERTAINMENT,
Being HUMOROUS, SENSATIONAL, DRAMATIC, PATHETIC, ORATORICAL, MUSICAL.

Athenæum Hall, Collins Street, Melbourne,

WEDNESDAY, MAY 11th, 1898.

MR. F. M. ALEXANDER'S

Dramatic & Elocutionary Recital.

PROGRAMME.

PART 1.

1. Pianoforte Solo ... "Andante De Salon 'Lucia De Lammermoor.'" ... *(G. Ascher o.p. 25.)*
   MR. G. BROMLEY.
2. Humorous Sketch ... "How he Proposed." ... ... *Anon*
   MISS EDITH TASCA-PAGE.
3. Song ... ... "The Cry of the Little Ones." ... ... *Adams*
   (By Special Request.)
   MISS LILIAN TWYCROSS.
4. Dramatic Sketch ... "Incident During the Indian Mutiny." ... ... *F. Poy*
   MR. F. M. ALEXANDER.
5. Violin Solo ... ... "Saltarello" ... ... *Papini*
   MISS GERTRUDE SUMMERHAYES.
   Accompanied by Madame Cecilia Summerhayes.
6. Pathetic Sketch... ... "Keeping His Word" ... ... *Anon*
   MISS EDITH TASCA-PAGE.
7. Humorous Sketch ... "The Clock Mystery." ... ... *Anon*
   MR. F. M. ALEXANDER.

INTERVAL FIVE MINUTES.

PART 2.

1. Song ... ... "Bid me to Love." ... ... *Tours*
   Violin Obligato by Miss Gertrude Summerhayes.
   MISS LILIAN TWYCROSS.
2. Dramatic Sketch... ... "The Midnight Charge." ... ...*Clement Scott*
   MR. F. M. ALEXANDER.
3. Humorous Scene from "The School for Scandal." { Lady Teazle ... ... MISS EDITH TASCA-PAGE. / Sir Peter Teazle ... ... MR. JAMES CATHCART.
4. Violin Solo ... ... "Nocturne in E Flat" ... ... *Chopin-Sarasate*
   MISS GERTRUDE SUMMERHAYES.
   Accompanied by Madame Cecilia Summerhayes.
5. Humorous Racing Sketch ... "The Amateur Rider." ... ... *Paterson*
   MR. F. M. ALEXANDER.

PIANO FROM MESSRS. CARNEGIE & SONS, ELIZABETH STREET.

Doors Open 7.30. Commence 8. Carriages 10.

HUGO FISCHER, Manager.

G. A. Green, Printer, M'Killop Street, Melbourne.

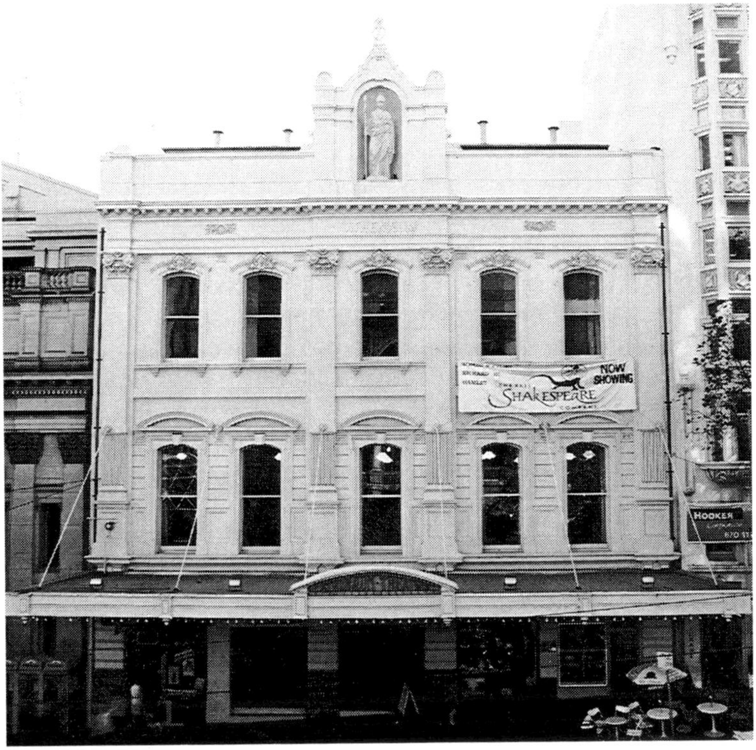

The Athenaeum, Collins Street, Melbourne (Courtesy of The Melbourne Athenaeum)

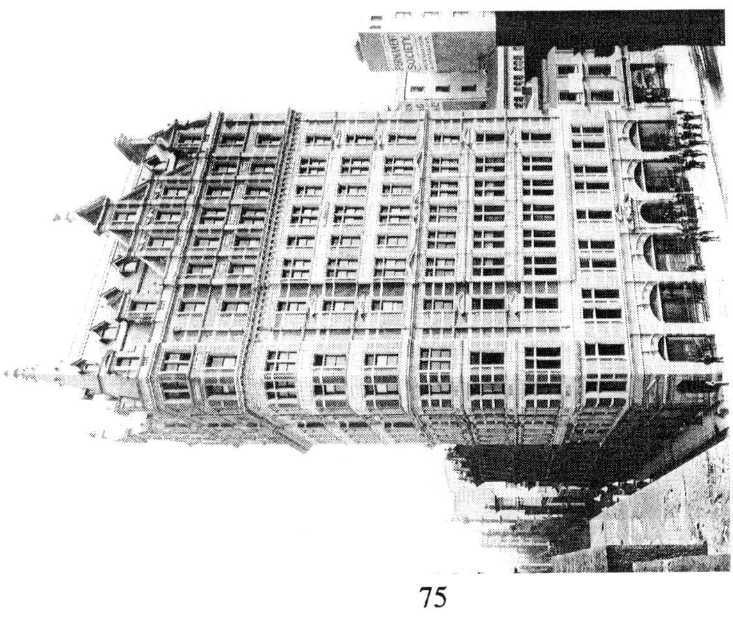

Australian Building, 49 Elizabeth Street, Melbourne
Opened 1889 Demolished 1981
(Courtesy of Royal Historical Society of Victoria)

Table Talk, a Melbourne general weekly newspaper with good theatre coverage reported, May 13th, 1898, *"Mr F. M. Alexander had the satisfaction of seeing a very large attendance at his dramatic and elocutionary recital on Wednesday evening, in the Athenaeum Hall. The welcome extended to him was hearty and encouraging, and each of his items was encored. As an elocutionist, Mr Alexander knows his business. He speaks the English language in a cultured, deliberate fashion that allows no slurring of words or dropping of final syllables. It is pleasing and satisfactory to listen to him. The wretched acoustic properties of the hall interfered with his success in the quieter passages of the recitations, but in narrative, declamation, and vigorous dialogue, Mr Alexander made effective use of his voice. 'An Incident of the Indian Mutiny', 'The Clock Mystery', 'The Midnight Charge', and 'The Amateur Rider' (also known as 'Kissing Cup's Race') covered a wide range of subject, and proved the reciter's ability - the last piece being the first in merit.*

"A pupil of Mr Alexander (Miss Edith Tasca-Page) recited two pieces, 'How he Proposed' and 'Keeping his Word', in a delicate sympathetic style, well-suited to drawing room entertainments. Miss Page has a very prepossessing appearance, and a pleasant even voice. A scene from 'The School for Scandal', by Mr James Cathcart and Miss Page took very well, and the audience greeted the only Sir Peter Teazle of Australia with enthusiasm. The violin playing of Miss Gertrude Summerhayes, and the singing of Miss Lilian Twycross, met with such favour that extra pieces had to be given. Mr G. Bromley opened the programme with a piano solo".

As he achieved success in his recitals, FM at the same time advertised his teaching methods. The Age, May 14th, 1898, *"New Methods in Speaking and Singing are imparted to students by Mr Alexander, Studio, 49 Elizabeth Street, who appeared with such great success at the Athenaeum Hall on Wednesday last."* Similarly, The Argus, July 2nd, 1898, *"Elocution, natural, imparted in theory and practice' the new methods. Mr Alexander, 49 Elizabeth St".*

With a fairly established reputation as a reciter in Melbourne, FM appeared in Adelaide at the Town Hall on July 22nd and 23rd, 1898, the advertisement for the second performance on July 23rd announcing, *"Positively Last Night, Owing to Forward Engagements, Positively Last Appearance of F. M. Alexander, the Famous Versatile Entertainer".*

The South Australian Register critique for the performance included the following, *"The second dramatic and elocutionary recital by Mr F. M. Alexander attracted an appreciative audience to the Town Hall on Friday evening, when a varied and interesting programme was presented. Mr Alexander gave a satisfactory rendering of those powerful lines 'Napoleon the*

Great' and fairly revelled in the humour of 'The Amateur Rider'. His rendering of 'Karl the Martyr' was dramatic and effective, 'The Clock Mystery', repeated by request, again exercised an unmistakable influence over the risible faculties of the audience, and 'The Midnight Charge' was a thoroughly satisfactory effort. With Miss Edith Tasca-Page he was heard in a humorous sketch from Tobin's comedy 'The Honeymoon' and an excerpt from 'The School for Scandal'. Miss Tasca-Page contributed a humorous sketch 'After Marriage', and infused considerable pathos into her rendering of the familiar recitation ~Keeping his Word', while her efforts in a dramatic sketch, 'Lasca', were thoroughly appreciated. Miss Gertrude Summerhayes is a violinist of considerable powers. She displays a capital tone, reliable intonation, and fine technique".

The above critique was appreciative but not all comments were quite so kind; *"Mr Alexander is a conscientious reciter, pleasing and natural in his style and gesture."*; *"being possesed of a voice mediocre in its quality, but excellent pronunciation, evident care in the study of his subjects, and a masterly knowledge of the art of elocution overcome this natural deficiency".*

On August 26th 1899 FM teamed up with Robert Young to present an evening of entertainment at the Athenaeum Hall based on the German Reed-Corney Grain repertory. Table Talk, September 8th, 1899, *"Mr F. M. Alexander in his natural and unaffected style gave two recitations, one The Death of Poor Jo (Dickens), the other, The Martyr, a most dreadful story. In each case he was encored and replied with humorous pieces".*

The Australasian (Melbourne weekly), September 2nd, 1899, under the heading Entertainments devoted a large space to expounding on the opportunity to present a German Reed-Corney Grain style of entertainment and to the actual performance, *"The enterprise of amusement caterers has not 'run' much of late to the drawingroom entertainment ...... Thousands of people who do not take their young fry to theatres, much less to music-halls...- are ready to support an entertainment of the German Reed pattern animated and humorous, yet circumspect, devoid of any element which could be detrimental to the schoolgirl, let alone the 'young person'".*

Thomas German Reed (1817 - 1888) was an English musician and entertainer, who played the violin and organ. From 1838 to 1851 he was musical director of the Haymarket Theatre, where he introduced good incidental music, overtures and entr'actes for the Shakespearean performances of Macready, the Keans (who later were to visit Australia) and the Cushmans. His wife was a prominent and sought-after performer as both actress and singer. In 1855 the Reeds began giving performances under the title of 'Mr and Mrs German Reed's Entertainment'. They became widely known in England.

The aim of their programmes was to provide good dramatic entertainment for the many people who, for various reasons, objected to the theatres.

After a few years the German Reeds were joined by several others, including their son Alfred German Reed and R. Corney Grain. Their repertory included operettas and pieces with texts by W. S. Gilbert and others. From about 1877 for a period of eighteen years Corney Grain and Alfred German Reed (the son of Thomas German Reed) produced most of the entertainment. A main feature of the entertainments were the musical sketches of Corney Grain which parodied the various European styles of singing.

The Australasian continued, *"Messrs. F. M. Alexander and Robert Young took possession of the Athenaeum Hall last Saturday, with an entertainment frankly imitative of the Reed-cum-Corney Grain performances, and they succeeded in pleasing a large audience. Mr Young has all the fine qualifications for success in this line of business. ..Mr Alexander's share in the entertainment consists of recitations, grave and gay. He is commendable both for what he does and what he avoids doing. He wisely makes no attempt at pieces requiring intensely dramatic or tragic power, such as would be selected by a Farirclough or a Montgomery. `Eugene Aram', `The Raven', `The Battle of Ivry', and so on, have been done so often by elocutionists with great command of vehemence and weird effect, that it is wasted labour now for performers more lightly equipped to essay them".*

The Athenaeum Hall, where FM chose to give recitals, has a long and fascinating history. The Melbourne Athenaeum, as it is called today, is the oldest public institution in Victoria. Its forerunner was a Mechanics Institute, founded in October 1839 when the colony of Victoria was only a few years old. During the 1840's a substantial two storey brick building was built in Collins Street in the Melbourne city centre, comprising hall, reading room, library and small museum. At this stage lighting at night was by candles, or lamp; the reading room was lit by candles which changed to gas light in the 1850's.

Over subsequent years there were many improvements and enlargement of facilities. In 1873 the Melbourne Mechanics Institution and School of Arts changed its name to the Melbourne Athenaeum. In 1887 after the new buildings had been completed a statue of Athena, goddess of the arts was placed on the building. By the 1890's there were well over one thousand members who made extensive use of the library and reading rooms. There was a large and smaller hall available for hire. Over the years the Athenaeum has undergone changes, partly brought about as new ways of entertainment such as film and TV altered the habits of the public. In 1989 the Institution celebrated its 150th birthday. The actual building is on the State's Register of Historic Buildings, and the facilities of the Melbourne Athenaeum today comprise a large library and two theatres.

Colleagues

Amongst the artists who appeared with FM at his recitations were Miss Edith Tasca-Page, Miss Lilian Twycross, Miss Gerturde Summerhayes, Madame Cecilia Summerhayes, Mr Robert Young and Mr James Cathcart.

Tasmanian born Edith Mary Page (1865 - 1938) was married in 1883 in St.David's Cathedral, Hobart to Mr Robert F. Young, a Civil Servant. In 1894, also in Hobart, Mrs R.Young took part in an FM recitation evening. Subsequently she performed with FM in Melbourne and Adelaide (1898) under the stage name Edith Tasca-Page. From 1900 to 1904 she was associated with both FM's recital and Shakespeare programs in Sydney and was also an elocution teaching colleague. She was widowed in 1910, and married FM in London in 1914.

Miss Lilian Twycross was an accomplished singer.She became a pupil of FM's and in 1898 her advertisements as a singing teacher appeared as follows, *"Miss Lilian Twycross. Singing Voice Cultivated. Thorough Training in Voice Production. Perfect System of Breathing. Reference kindly permitted to the Bishop of Melbourne, Sir John Madden, F. M. Alexander Esq., Dr Rankin, and other influential citizens. Testimonials. Glen's, Collins St. Monday and Thursday Afternoons ".* (Sir John Madden was also a pupil of FM.) This style of lay-out for her advertisements seemed to be used consistently, for a time.

Miss Gertrude Summerhayes came from a highly gifted musical family. She arrived in Australia when only a few years old, with her mother and brother. Her mother Madame Cecilia Summerhayes, was a noted British pianist who was chosen by the Brinsmead piano firm in England to demonstrate and give recitals using their instruments, which were on display at the Sydney International Exhibition of 1879. The boat journey out to Australia was so terrible that Madame Summerhayes decided not to return to England. She taught for a while in Sydney, then the family was briefly in Tasmania and New Zealand (at least the boat trips were not so long as England to Australia), then finally they settled in Melbourne. The Summerhayes family became involved in Melbourne's artistic life. Mother, and daughter Gertrude, a fine violinist, played at many musical functions. Madame Summerhayes accompanied Mrs Helen Armstrong on a number of occasions; this was before Mrs Armstrong went overseas, and became known as Dame Nellie Melba.

Mr Robert Young was associated with FM's performances in Hobart, Melbourne and later in Sydney. His work reflected the Reed-Corney Grain influence, he was talented in various artistic areas - piano, mime, comic, song and composition.

Mr James Cathcart was a long-time resident and respected actor in Australia. His sister, Fanny Cathcart was the more prominent member of the family, who first came to Australia in 1855 as the leading lady for the Australian tour by G. V. Brooke. She subsequently toured Australia a number of times, then settled here. She died in Melbourne in 1880. James Cathcart had been performing in Australia since the 1860s. He became well established here. In the 1890's he was giving Dramatic Interpretation and Elocution lessons in Melbourne. There is also an interesting advertisement, October 7th, 1893, for an event at the Theatre Royal, announced as a Grand Football Demonstration. It was to be an entertainment and presentation of trophies night for the end of the football season in Melbourne. A big event, as Australian Rules Football is the dominant winter sport in Melbourne. There were representatives from twelve clubs, including South Adelaide (from South Australia). The entertainment programme included Mr James F. Cathcart, the Popular Actor and Elocutionist who was to recite 'Australia's Game, Football', by Mr Pat Finn.

The critique for James Cathcart's performance as Sir Peter Teazle, for one of FM's recital programmes in 1898, stated, *"the audience greeted the only Sir Peter Teazle* (James Cathcart) *of Australia with enthusiasm"*. An indication of the respect accorded him.

Clients

The people who came to FM for lessons were from a wide range of Melbourne society. The art of eloquent speech in public speaking was much admired, and for the clergy, politicians or lawyers this skill was a necessity. There were no microphones then, this technology being a twentieth century development.

What follows are thumbnail sketches of a cross-section of FM's Melbourne pupils and supporters, and extracts from some of their references given to FM when he transferred his teaching to Sydney in 1900. These references mostly appear in FM's Sydney advertisements for his teaching methods and in the small treatise which he printed and made available to prospective pupils.

THE CLERGY

Soon after FM had established himself in Melbourne as a vocal art teacher he was approached by the Baptist Theological College and asked if he would take elocution classes for the students for the ministry. This was not a new idea, a previous teacher had already taught Elocution there. FM agreed to the request. The College Principal's Report of 1897 states, *"Our students have been under the training of Mr Alexander for the production of the voice and for breathing. Improvement has been noted both at the sermon class and by worshippers at services conducted by our men"*. It is not clear as to how long FM continued taking these classes. In 1899 - 1900 a new Elocution teacher, a lady, was appointed to the position, the first lady tutor appointed by the Baptist College.

Certainly FM's teaching at the Baptist Theological College was appreciated. When he went to work in Sydney (1900), a reference was given to him by the Honorary Secretary of the College, H. Sumner Martin. Mr Martin was also a long-serving Legal Adviser for the Baptist Church. He wrote to FM, *"Not only are the students very pleased with the trouble which you have taken with them, but the committee are gratified to learn from those who hear them regularly that there has been a considerable improvement owing to your teaching"*.

The Rev. E Handel Jones was a Congregational Minister who trained at the Bristol Institute, England (1871 - 1873). Then after some years in the Ministry at North Petherton, Somerset, he came to Melbourne in 1887. He was in charge of parishes in various parts of Victoria, then went to the Congregational Church in Davey Street, Hobart, Tasmania in 1908, where he remained until 1915. Records of his further whereabouts were not available. He evidently thought highly of the lessons he had with FM, as is shown by the following,
"I have pleasure in bearing my testimony to the value of the breathing method as taught by you. Its effects on my general health are most grafitying - inspiring one with hope for the future. Breathing, once a difficulty, has now, after a few lessons only, imparted to me new life, enabling me to walk a greater distance with less fatigue. So perfect is the equilibrium and general control of the body secured by your method that going up and down stairs, which I once dreaded is now performed with ease. If the `breath is the life', the right use of breathing power is of paramount importance. I regard your process of breathing as the most natural, philosophic and effective I have ever tried. What others teach in theory, you simplify and embody in practice, placing Nature's principles within reach of all. Your system deserves to be universally known - not least to vocalists and public speakers and all suffering with throat and chest affections".

A member of the Carmelites, Rev. Prior Thomas P. Kelly was another who had had his fair share of throat trouble. Prior Kelly (1854 - 1926), had attended the Catholic University in Dublin and was a man of great erudition, a first class classical scholar and mathematician. He was in Melbourne as a Prior of the Carmelites from 1894 to 1904. He wrote about his lessons with FM,

"I am really sorry that we, in Melbourne, will lose you through your leaving for Sydney. I have never known a teacher of voice-production, etc., so successful, or one who so fully accomplishes what he professes as you. 'Tis to my mind lamentable that such wide-spread neglect in voice-training and breathing should exist. Our heads of schools, if only in the interests of their pupils' throats and general health, should insist on every teacher understanding something of the principles underlying voice-training. Personally, I am under deep obligations to you for help which, if I had received long ago, would have saved many a miserable hour of throat trouble. I have never known a case entrusted to your care to fail".

A Presbyterian Minister, the Rev. John Vance wrote,
"I went to you wholly ignorant of the science of voice-production and very imperfect in the art. You soon convinced me that my estimation of my ignorance was not exaggerated. You taught me the principles of proper breathing, the laws of inflection, modulation, etc., of the voice. A change of voice and the much-needed improvement of delivery of sermons was noted by my congregation in about two months' time, and was appreciated. I am now less tired after my day's work than I was formerly after any morning service. You gave me sufficient knowledge to enable me to continue my practice privately, and my hope is that some day I may attain something of the perfection of my teacher. I regret much you are leaving Melbourne. We need a few such voice trainers here".

THE DOCTORS

FM was able to establish a rapport with a number of influential doctors, first in Melbourne, then later in Sydney. Some doctors were FM's pupils, others gave him patient referrals.

Dr Charles Bage (1859-1930) was born in the colony of Victoria. He attended Melbourne Grammar School where his all-round ability in both scholastic study and sport led to his becoming head prefect in 1876. He went on to study medicine at Melbourne University, graduating in Bachelor of Medicine and Bachelor of Surgery in 1881 and Doctor of Medicine in 1884. A keen interest in languages and literature led him to continue academic studies and graduate from the University with an M.A. in 1887. Dr. Bage worked initially at the Melbourne Hospital then commenced private practice in South Yarra where he continued until 1923. (In the 1890's Dr. Bage was FM Alexander's doctor. In the latter part of that period he had lessons from FM and sent a number of his patients to FM as pupils.)

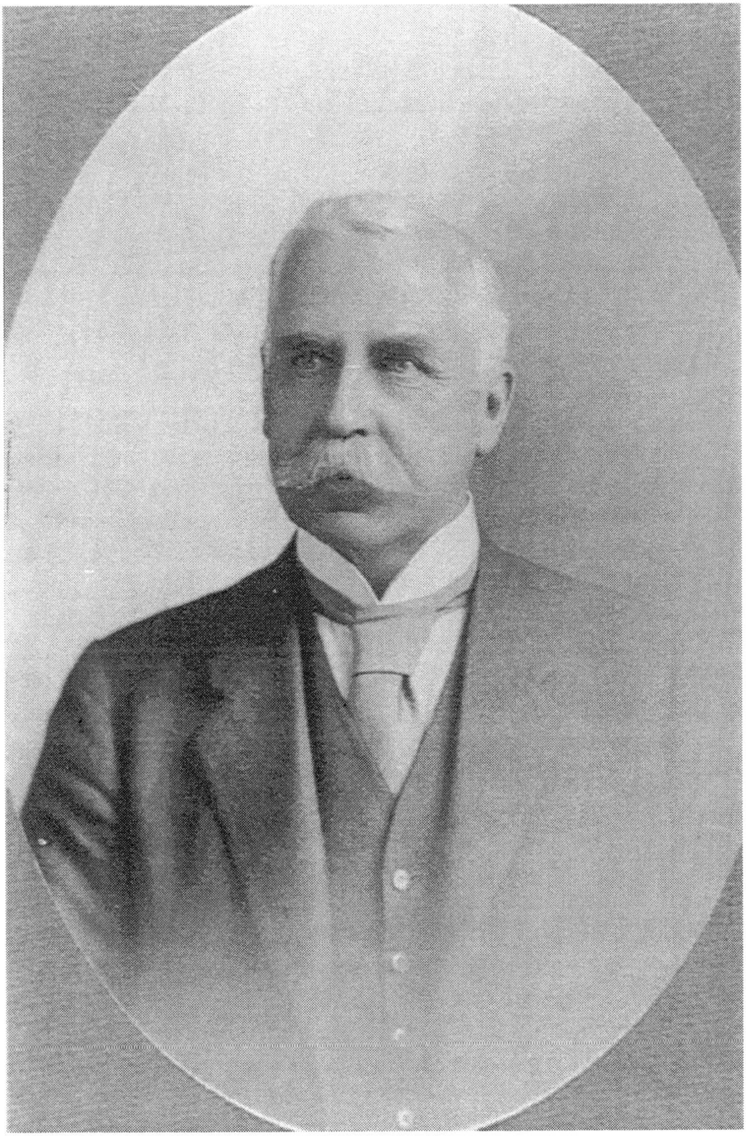

Dr Bage (Courtesy of the family of Dr Bage)

Apart from his private practice Dr. Bage maintained a strong association with the Melbourne University Medical Faculty, as examiner and lecturer. For many years he was closely connected with the St. John Ambulance Association and the Australian Red Cross Society, holding executive positions in both organisations. He took a keen interest in public health and was a member of the Council of the Australian Health Society from 1901. Dr. Bage was particularly interested in the study of tuberculosis and spent much time in alerting people to the causes and prevention of this disease. He gave numerous public lectures on diverse aspects of medical science. On October 1st, 1898 Dr. Bage gave a lecture on Consumption (TB) at the Assembly Hall, Melbourne for the Australian Health Society. (In December 1903 in Sydney FM published an article in the Daily Telegraph entitled, the Prevention and Cure of Consumption.) In this era the topic of Consumption was in the forefront of public health matters.

Dr. Bage had wide community interests. He was on the Council of his old school, Melbourne Grammar; he was a member of the Felton Bequest Committee from its inception in 1904 and Chairman from 1910 to 1930. This Trust, which still continues, has been most beneficial to Victoria, assisting many charities, and also, through its purchase of private works of art for the National Gallery of Victoria, playing a role of inestimable value for that institution.

Dr. Bage had a wide circle of friends and associates in Melbourne, including Dr. Alexander Leeper (who was to have contact with FM in 1908 in London). The obituary in the Medical Journal of Australia for February 7th, 1931 gives evidence of the esteem in which Dr. Bage was held by his colleagues.

When FM moved to Sydney in 1900 Dr.Bage wrote to him expressing regret that he was transferring to Sydney and wishing him all success there. Dr Bage continued; *"If it is any use to you to do so, please refer to me as one of your pupils. After a course of lessons from you, I am fully convinced that your confidence in the correctness of your methods is abundantly justified. The exercises you give not only improve the tone of the voice, but also lessen the strain of loud or continued speaking. In addition, they tend to benefit the general health by inducing good habits of breathing".*

The above was not the last correspondence between Dr. Bage and FM After he went to England in 1904, FM sent Dr. Bage a copy of his first book, Man's Supreme Intelligence. Dr. Bage replied as follows:

South Yarra,
Melbourne,
Jan. 12th, 1911.

Dear Mr Alexander,
Many thanks for your book which I have read with great interest. Your essay makes out a good case for conscious control — for conscious inhibition of faulty muscular habits; but it is inevitable that when it comes to practical application of methods of training every teacher of good quality will have some positive ways of his own for which he will claim special excellence.

Even judgment by results is not an infallible guide to the relative values of different methods, for as you know there is so much difference between different pupils at the start. The teacher's greatest need and greatest recommendation is confidence in his own way, and an enthusiastic readiness for good results and these qualities I am convinced have gone far towards making your own undoubted success. Your quickness in clearing respiratory and oral faults and in correcting them is the result of practical experience rather than of scientific induction, but I congratulate you in maintaining the keen interest in your work that induces you to stand back from it now and then and generalise philosophically about it.

Many thanks for the postcards you have sent me now and then. What a delight to be within such easy distance of foreign lands. Please give my kind remembrances to all — and believe me

Yours sincerely,
Charles Bage

Reprinted by kind permission of the family of Dr. Charles Bage

Dr Augustus Kenny (1863 - 1946), born in England of Irish parents; the family emigrated to Melbourne in 1870. A medical graduate from Melbourne University, Dr Kenny served medicine with distinction for many decades. Apart from this major professional contribution to both the community of Victoria and the medical profession, Dr Kenny had wide sporting and artistic interests and supported many charitable movements. He explored new ideas and was willing, where appropriate, to refer his patients to FM, *"Have much pleasure in stating that certain patients of mine, with throat ailments, have been markedly benefited by lessons in breathing and voice production given by Mr F. Matthias Alexander".*

Dr Donald S. MacColl (1862 - 1938) was born in Inverness, Scotland. His professional studies were in medicine and he came to Australia about 1890. In 1891 he gave medical aid to the students at the Baptist Theological College in Melbourne. He was widely respected in Melbourne. As well as his medical work he was a lay preacher for the Baptist Church. Dr MacColl wrote to FM, *"I feel confident that your methods are excellent, and will do all in my power to further your interests. The Bearer, Rev.-, is suffering from a throat affection. I have suggested to him he should see you, as I am confident you can help him".*

Another doctor who supported FM's work was Dr. Walter Balls-Headley (1841 - 1918). He was English born and studied medicine in London. He emigrated first to Queensland then moved to Melbourne in the 1870's and was elected physician to the Alfred Hospital in 1876. In 1878 he was appointed to the Women's Hospital, a position he held with distinction until 1900. Dr.Balls-Headley was one of the leading gynaecologists in Melbourne. He lectured at the Medical Faculty, Melbourne University and held prominent positions in a number of medical organisations. In the early 1900's he returned to England for a short time then retirement was spent in British Columbia.

THE LAWYERS AND POLITICIANS

Sir John Madden (1844 - 1918), came with his family from Ireland to Melbourne in 1857. Prior to coming here the family had lived for three years in London and young John had spent two years of this time attending school at Beauchamps, France. After graduating in law from Melbourne University in 1865, he practised law here for many years, rising to the position of Chief Justice of Victoria in 1893. For several years he was a member of the Victorian Parliament and he kept his links with Melbourne University through being on the University Council. From 1897 until his death in 1918, Sir John was Chancellor of the University. He obviously had strong views about standards of speech and the value of Mr Alexander's work as is evidenced by the following comments.

This reprint is from The Herald (Melbourne newspaper), *"When the Chief Justice of the colony is prompted to say that there is a danger of Australia being `damned with small voices', when it is quite a rare thing to find a witness in a court of law who can speak up and make himself heard, when one's ears are offended by barristers who have voices which creak and grate like rusty saws, when our public platforms are largely occupied by men who have not the smallest conception of speaking - we are inclined to think that the services of a man like Mr Alexander ought to be in constant and eager demand. It is an entirely wrong idea that it is only singers who need their voices trained. There are probably not a dozen men in Parliament who know how to use their voices; yet members of Parliament are constantly addressing public meetings and using their voices. And in sheer ignorance of how to speak, they either bawl or mutter - suggesting either the bellowing of the bull of Bashan, or the* *feeble bleating of a consumptive sheep. And then again, how few parsons know how to read. By all such people a man like Mr F. M. Alexander should be regarded as a friend and counsellor. It is the aim of all right-thinking people to improve their intellects. The training of their voices is as important, and the study connected with it necessitates the use and cultivation of the intellectual faculties".*

Sir William Harrison Moore (1867 - 1935). Born in London, he graduated in law, first from Cambridge then the University of London. He was a fine scholar and in 1892 he arrived in Melbourne to take up the post of Professor of Law at Melbourne University. This youthful professor was to serve the University, and Australia, with distinction. After he retired from the University in 1927 he continued with legal work, being involved with the League of Nations as an Australian delegate. He had also contributed much in the area of constitutional law and was an acknowledged authority with regard to the Constitution for the new Federation of the Colonies, which became the Commonwealth of Australia in 1901.

Professor W. Harrison Moore wrote to FM, *"I have great pleasure in expressing my high apprecitaion of the pains you took during the course of elocution lessons which I have had from you. I am very sensible of the value of your instruction as a means of economising strength in what all who have to practise it know to be the very arduous work of public speaking, and before I heard of your intended departure from Melbourne I was urging others to seek your aid. My regret is that your departure for Sydney will prevent me from continuing a course which I ought to have taken years ago".*

David C. Rees (1847 - 1907) like many other Victorians of those times, came to Victoria as a youngster. Welsh born, he attended Melbourne University and was admitted to practise as a barrister and solicitor in Victoria in 1877. He held high office in the Government, being the Chief Examiner of Titles in the Land Titles Office, Melbourne. He was very involved with the Baptist Church and was for some time, Treasurer of the Baptist Theological College of Victoria.

David Rees wrote to FM, *"Having seen your treatise, I decided to take your course of `breathing lessons'. I had some knowledge of the theory, obtained by reading, but I found that your lessons supplied very satisfactorily what was lacking in the books published on the subject. I can, therefore, testify to your ability in communicating to pupils the knowledge that you possess, and can state that I found very little difficulty in acquiring the art of proper breathing after obtaining your explanation and following out the course of PRACTICAL lessons you gave. I found, too, a very distinct advantage - SO FAR AS HEALTH WAS CONCERNED - from practising the method of breathing which you prescribed".*

Sir Arthur Robinson (1872 - 1945). Melbourne born, he studied law at Melbourne University, then built up a successful legal practice. At various times he was a member of the Victorian Parliament, and the Commonwealth Parliament. Sir Arthur had extensive commercial and financial interests, and took a keen interest in sport. He wrote to FM, *"I can see the great benefits I have derived from your teaching, not only as regards speaking, but also my general health".*

Consolidation and Change

FM had developed a substantial teaching practice in Melbourne since he first started in 1896. He was later joined by his brother, Albert Reddon Alexander (known as AR) and his sister Amy. Both worked as assistants to FM in Australia although their work lacks documentation. Certainly AR's presence in Melbourne made it possible for FM to leave the city and to travel to other areas, spreading knowledge of his methods.

Bendigo, a city one hundred and fifty kilometres north of Melbourne, was a hive of activity during the gold rush, and still is a main centre for the northern parts of Victoria. The Bendigo Advertiser, October 21st, 1899, carried the following advertisement,

"TO SINGERS AND SPEAKERS TO SINGERS AND SPEAKERS The Three Important Acts neglected in the cultivation of the Singing and Speaking Voice in Australasia are - Full Chest Breathing, Proper Manipulation, Correct Formation of the Resonance Cavities, and without them the human voice cannot possibly be thorougly developed or used to the best advantage in speech and song. Singing and speaking should not be attempted until the student has thoroughly mastered these arts. They would then become proficient singers and speakers in one quarter the usual time, and avoid the majority of the difficulties they must otherwise encounter.

"MR F. M. ALEXANDER, who has imparted the new methods in vocal use in Melbourne during the past four years will visit Bendigo every Wednesday to receive students for a course of study, and may be interviewed at ...... Private Hotel, near railway station, on that day. The first lesson of the course will be given on Wednesday next. Intending students should communicate with Mr Alexander at his studio, Australian Buildings, 49 Elizabeth Street, Melbourne, where treatise on voice culture may be obtained free by sending your address. Mr Alexander is prepared to receive a limited number of students for Elocution, Natural Dramatic Training, Cultivation of Singing and Speaking Voice by the New Methods, Full Chest Breathing. Invaluable to singers and speakers, and those with weak chests. Breathing gymnastics. Cure for Throat Troubles arising from imperfect vocal use. Singers or speakers".

FM moved to Sydney in early 1900, and the studio he had rented in Melbourne in the Australian Building became vacant. AR did not continue the Melbourne practice for long; in February 1901 he enlisted in the Fifth (Mounted Rifles) Contingent, part of the Australian Military Contingents to the War in South Africa (the Boer War). AR, who was twenty-six years of age, listed his occupation as stockman. After the war duty in South Africa, the Fifth Contingent returned to Melbourne in April 1902, and was then disbanded.

In 1904 there was again an Alexander listed as a tenant on the seventh floor of the Australian Building at 49 Elizabeth Street. It was AR, sharing studio space with Miss Lilian Twycross, who was an important figure in the unfolding of the Alexander work in the early days in Australia. It is interesting to note that in 1904 AR listed himself as an elocutionist, but from 1905 until he went to England in 1911, he put alongside his name, 'breathing and medical exercise'. But in another part of the same directory, he still keeps the label, 'elocutionist'. About the same time that AR went to England, his sister Amy went too. She later married there. A daughter Marjorie became a teacher of FM Alexander's work and wife to Dr Wilfred Barlow, a prominent British doctor, Alexander teacher and researcher.

In October 1907 AR Alexander applied to become a teacher under the Registration of Teachers and Schools Act 1905. The Teachers and Schools Registration Board received thousands of applications in the first few years of its existence. This registration was for people who were not in the State Government Education Department (see chapter 12.) AR was a private teacher with his own studio, but registration would give more status. His application form stated he had been teaching Elocution and Physical Culture in private practice since 1896. (This would have been interrupted by his Boer War service.) The classification AR sought was as a secondary teacher of the following special subjects: Elocution and Physical Culture, Respiration, Deportment, Gesture etc. Under academic qualifications he stated he was a student of Anatomy and Physiology under Professor Young of Hunter St., Sydney (see latter part of Chapter 13.) AR said his teaching experience extended over eleven years in Sydney and Melbourne and during that time students and patients had been recommended to him by Drs. Kenny, Maudsley, Morrison, Bage, Hamilton, Seelenmeyer and others of Melbourne, and Drs. Brady, Nolan, Clubbe and J. W. Stewart McKay of Sydney. AR was granted registration and was to have further contact with the Board.

Some details have already been given in this chapter re Dr. Kenny and Dr. Bage. Dr. Adolphe F. Seelenmeyer (1855-1922) was born in England and came to Melbourne in the mid 1870's to work as a pharmacist alongside his brother. In the 1880's he gained medical qualifications in Brussels and Edinburgh then returned to Melbourne where he established a private medical practice and was on the staff at Prince Henry's Hospital.

Sir Henry Carr Maudsley (1859-1944) was born in Yorkshire, completed his education in London graduating with first class honours in medicine in 1881. After further medical study and experience Dr. Maudsley emigrated to Melbourne in 1888, obtaining an appointment at the Alfred Hospital. From 1903 until the outbreak of WWI he was on the staff of the Royal Melbourne Hospital. From 1908-21 (except for War service 1914-19) Dr. Maudsley was a lecturer in theory and practice of medicine at Melbourne University. He served with distinction in WWI, reaching the rank of Colonel and being honoured with a Knighthood. His appointments included senior physician 1st Australian General Hospital, Australian Imperial Force, later consulting physician at A.I.F. Headquarters, London. In 1919 Sir Henry Maudsley returned to Melbourne and resumed private practice. At the height of his powers he was regarded as a fine clinical teacher at the Royal Melbourne Hospital and one of Melbourne's leading physicians, with a particular interest in neurology.

Apart from registering teachers the Teachers and Schools Registration Board set the standards and the syllabus. The following are extracts from Minutes of the Teachers and Registration Board Meetings re Elocution, a subject over which the Board subsequently relinquished control.

23/09/1907: *"It was further resolved that the minimum literary qualification to be accepted by the Board from Teachers of Elocution would be the Senior Public Examination (English)."*

14/10/1907: *"The Registrar stated that Miss Godwin Smith, Mr Howlett Ross and Mr A R Alexander had consented to act on the advisory committee on Elocution. Miss Henderson and Dr.Leeper were appointed as members of the Committee.*
Dr.Leeper to act as Chairman."

12/11/1907: *"The reports of the advisory committees appointed to draw up the requirements to be demanded from persons applying for registration as teachers of Elocution, of Book-keeping, of Shorthand and Typewriting were considered by the Board.*

"In connection with teachers of Elocution it was decided to amend the committee's recommendation by inserting the words "the elementary principles of" before the words "the anatomy, hygiene, and physiology of the vocal organs" and "respiration."

"On the motion of Dr Leeper and Miss Henderson it was resolved that the following requirements for teachers of elocution be adopted by the Board: -

TEACHERS OF SPECIAL SUBJECTS

REQUIREMENTS FOR REGISTRATION UNDER THE HEADING OF "FITNESS TO TEACH."

ELOCUTION.

1. Any person may be registered as a Teacher of the Special Subject of Elocution who applies for registration prior to 1st January, 1908, and who fulfils the following requirements:-

(i) Has passed a written examination satisfactory to the Board in the Subject of English on the same lines and of the same standard as the Junior Public Examination of the University of Melbourne, but omitting any prescribed Text Books;

(ii) Has passed a written examination satisfactory to the Board in the General Principles of Elocution (Text Book recommended - Hill's "Oratorical Trainer"); (See chapters 7,9.)

(iii) Has passed to the satisfaction of the Board a practical test in the knowledge of and power of teaching sound methods of respiration and articulation: and

(iv) Has passed to the satisfaction of the Board a practical test in reading and delivery.

2. After the 1st January, 1908, any person may be registered as a Teacher of the Special Subject of Elocution who fulfils the following requirements: -

(i) Has passed in English at the Senior Public Examination of the University of Melbourne, or some examination in English of equivalent stand; and

(ii) Has passed an examination satisfactory to the Board in the knowledge of the competency to teach -

(a) The elementary principles of the Anatomy, Hygiene, and Physiology of the Vocal Organs;
(b) The elementary principles of Respiration;
(c) Thorough Voice Production (including Articulation, Enunciation, Pronunciation, Correct Emphasis, Modulation); and
(d) Deportment (Gesture, Delivery, Attitude).

(The Examination to be mainly Practical.)"

21/02/1910: *"The following committee was appointed to draw up the details of arrangements for the testing of candidates for registration as Teachers of Elocution : -*
Dr. Leeper (Chairman), Miss Henderson, Dr. Harvey Sutton,
Dr Mary Booth and Mr Hanson."

14/03/1910: *"The Report of the Committee on Teachers of Elocution was considered by the Board. It was decided to adopt the following requirements for the registration of Teachers of Elocution : -*

Teachers and Schools Registration Board

TEACHERS OF SPECIAL SUBJECTS.

REQUIREMENTS FOR REGISTRATION UNDER THE HEADING OF "FITNESS TO TEACH."

ELOCUTION.

1. Any person may be registered as a Teacher of the Special Subject of Elocution who

(i) Has passed in English at the Senior Public Examination of the University of Melbourne, or some examination in English of equivalent standard; and

(ii) Has passed an examination satisfactory to the Board in the knowledge of and competency to teach -
(a) The elementary principles of the Anatomy, and of the Physiology of the Vocal Organs;
(b) The Hygiene of the Vocal and Respiratory Organs;
(c) The elementary principles of Respiration;
(d) Phonetics and Voice Production (including the treatment of defects of speech, such as stammering, etc.); and
(e) Interpretation.

NOTE; - The Examination under Sub-Section (ii) will be mainly Practical.

2. Any person may be registered as a Teacher of the Special Subject of Elocution who holds some qualification determined by the Board to be of equivalent standard to the qualifications set forth in Section 1.

BOOKS RECOMMENDED

SECTION 1 (ii) (a) -
As much as is contained in
Voice Production in Singing and Speaking - Mills (Curwen & Sons);

Or any of the following books -
Voice Training (Hulbert);
Voice, Song, and Speech (Brown and Behnke);
(See chapter 9.)
On Musical Education and Voice Culture (Bach).

(Special attention is drawn to the Physiology of Fatigue).

SECTION 1 (ii) (b) & (c) -

As much as is contained in the following sections of

Voice, Song, and Speech (Brown and Behnke) - "The Hygienic Aspect of the Vocal apparatus," "Voice Cultivation (Breathing and Attack,)" "The Daily Life of the Voice-User," "The Ailments of the Voice-User," "Defects of Speech - Stammering and Stuttering."

SECTION 1 (ii) (d) -
As much as is contained in

The Science of Speech (Dumville); and
Voice Training (Hulbert);

Or any of the following books -

The Pronunciation of English (Jones);
Elementary Phonetics (Scholle and Smith);
Elements of Phonetics (Rippmann);
The Sounds of Spoken English (Rippmann).

SECTION 1 (ii) (e) -
As much as is contained in ______

The Voice and Spiritual Education (Hiram Corson); and Essay on "The Study of Literature" (John Morley).

TEACHING OF ENGLISH -

The Teaching of English (Roberts and Barker);
" " " " *(Chubb)*
" " " " *(Carpenter);*
" " " " *(Baker and Scott).*

NOTE: - Candidates are recommended to study the best exponents of the arts of Public Speaking and Elocution."

10/6/1913: "That the following recommendation of the Registration Committee in regard to candidates for registration as Teachers of Elocution be adopted namely:

After 1st January 1914, candidates desiring registration as Teachers of Elocution must undergo the following course of training : -

(a) To study elementary Psychology, general method, and, especially, the method of English;
(b) To spend at least 80 hours in the observation and practice of teaching English, 60 hours of which should be spent in a primary school, and 20 hours in a secondary school.
(The motion was carried) "

2/09/1919: *"That a further effort be made to secure the registration of all teachers of physical culture and voice production."*

1/10/1919: *"The Report of the Committee appointed to draw up a memorandum to the Minister urging the registration of Teachers of Physical Culture was adopted by the Council. It was decided not to ask for the registration of Teachers of Elocution and Voice Production for the present."*

MISS LILIAN TWYCROSS

Miss Lilian Twycross (1874-1943) studied singing in Melbourne in the early 1890's. She then became a successful singing teacher and a fine contralto. She combined teaching and performance, her concert work extending well beyond Melbourne. Miss Twycross was one of FM's early pupils, and showed such understanding of the principles of his work that in 1898 FM wrote her the following reference,

" Dear Miss Twycross,

You should command success in the profession you have chosen, as you are capable of teaching Voice Production, Breathing, &c.

You possess the artistic sympathetic temperament, and should be equally successful from the aesthetic standpoint, as from the practical.
Feb. 1898. (signed) F. MATTHIAS ALEXANDER".

A second letter of appreciation was sent by FM to Miss Twycross at the end of 1898.

" As it is now the end of the second year you have assisted at my studio, I feel duty bound to send you this special acknowledgement of the valuable services you have rendered. I trust that I shall have your help during 1899. I assure you the splendid results of your labours are thoroughly appreciated by the students and myself."

An advertisement of that time by Miss Twycross has already been quoted.

After 1900 when FM went to Sydney and AR to the Boer War, Miss Twycross was for a time the only teacher in Melbourne of FM's methods as applied to speaking and singing. She advertised as follows,

" TO SINGERS and SPEAKERS
THE HUMAN VOICE MANAGED by MUSCLE ACTION.
Mr F. M. ALEXANDER, Vocal and Dramatic Studio, Sydney, writes: -
"Miss Lilian Twycross, for three years Chief Assistant at my studio, is the only certificated teacher of my methods applied to the speaking and singing voice in Melbourne," Perfect system of breathing (full-chest), invaluable to voice users, and those with weak chests. Throat Troubles, Hoarseness, Breaks Rapidly Removed. Every lesson illustrates a principle; every principle has a practical application.
Australian-Buildings, Elizabeth Street".

Later when FM was in London (from 1904) Miss Twycross advertised,

" *SINGING and SPEAKING. - Voice managed by MUSCLE ACTION, perfect BREATHING method, which prevents gasping, raising shoulders, taking air through mouth, throat troubles, hoarseness rapidly removed, Miss Lilian Twycross (certified pupil of Mr F. M. Alexander, London), Australian-bldgs., Elizabeth-st. Write for treatise, free".*

From 1904 until 1910 Miss Twycross shared teaching studios with AR Alexander on the seventh floor of the Australian Building, 49 Elizabeth Street. From 1910, Miss Twycross taught singing at Presbyterian Ladies' College, a leading Melbourne girls school.

The small advertisement detailed above, when FM was in London, stated at the end, *"Write for treatise, free."* This treatise is here printed in full. It no doubt had FM's approval and much of the wording indicates that they probably collaborated in the writing of it. FM himself had printed a small treatise about his methods in 1898, to publicize his methods. This is no longer extant. What follows would almost certainly bear a close resemblance to the long lost 1898 FM treatise.

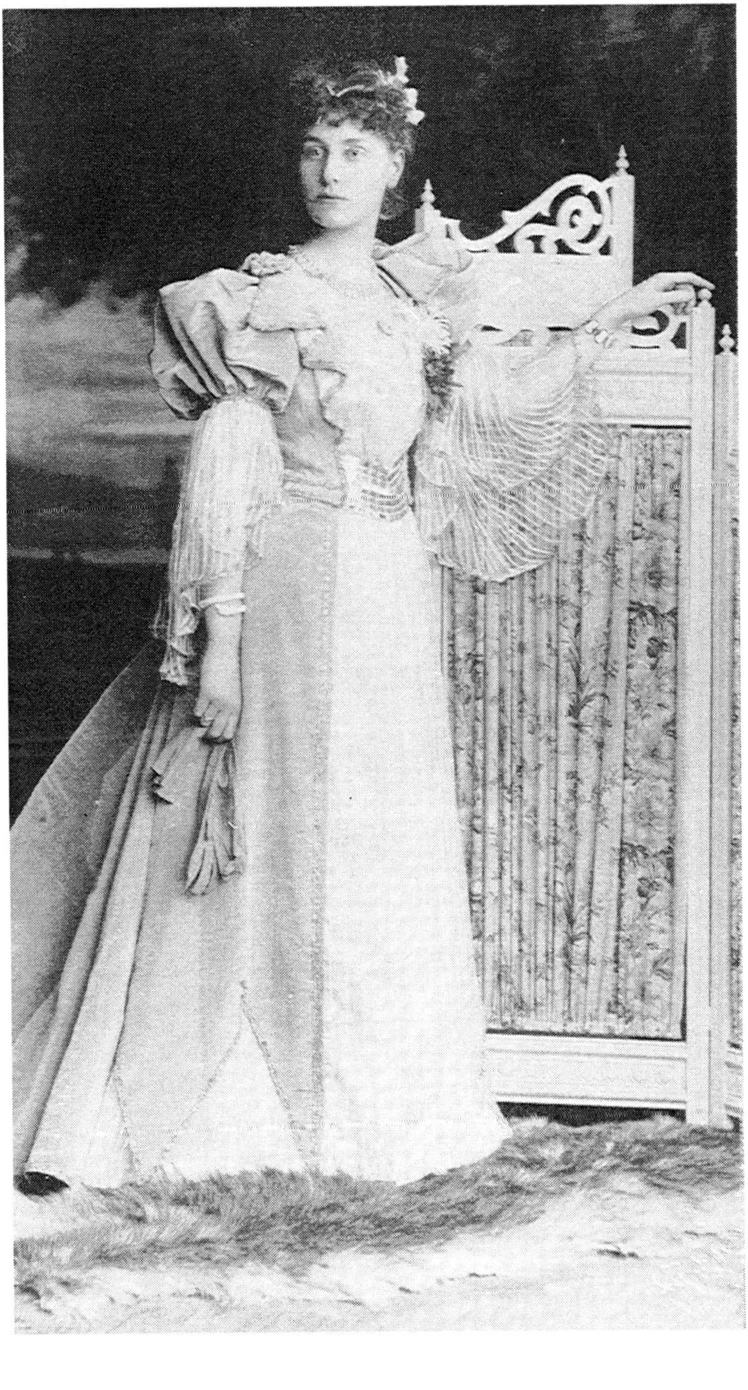

Miss Lilian Twycross (Courtesy of Mrs. E. Twycross Butler)

With Miss Lilian Twycross's Compliments.

... The ...

Cultivation and Development

OF THE

Human Voice

FOR

Singing

and

Speaking.

FULL-CHEST BREATHING.

CULTIVATION AND DEVELOPMENT OF THE HUMAN VOICE FOR SINGING AND SPEAKING

As Bach and other authorites state, only that method is correct which renders singing and speaking more and more easy, and makes it a pleasure to the voice-user and to those listening to him - "a consummation devoutly to be wish'd," but how attained? Primarily, by acquiring control, skilful manipulation, and an economical distribution of the motor-element - breath.

The fact that not one singer or speaker in a thousand knows how to breathe correctly proves the lack of knowledge existing relating to the above arts, which are indispensable to **Voice Culture.** As air is essential to the production of voice, the ability to inhale breath with the **whole chest** is of vital importance.

FULL-CHEST BREATHING AND PROPER MANIPULATION

must be the studies first mastered by the singer or speaker to ensure the successful **production** or **building** of the voice. This the false methods commonly imparted in Australasia, and also in most countries outside of the leading art centres of the Old World, do not admit of - the systems most in evidence among us being clavicular, costal and diaphragmatic breathing, neither of which admit of the expansion of the full chest, or the ability to supply the lungs with sufficient air through the **nostrils.** Mouth-breathing is then resorted to to obtain the necessary amount of air for singing and speaking. Mouth-breathing is injurious both from a vocal and hygienic standpoint, for the air, laden with impurities, comes in direct contact with the mucous membrane, causing inflammation and irritation, if not actual disease.

On the other hand, the nostrils are provided with a natural filter, enabling them to cast off all impurities. Inhaling through the nostrils also aids deep breathing, for the air, being more concentrated, exercises a greater pressure and descends deeper. It is admitted by the highest authorities that on the ability to economise the air in the important task of **exhalation** depends the strength, flexibility and sustaining power of the voice. As **Sir Morell Mackenzie** quaintly expresses it, *"The vocal cords must use the breath as Jacob did the angel with whom he wrestled - they must not suffer it to depart till it has blessed them"*. Control over the breath in exhaling is not possible when the false methods before referred to are employed. The controlling muscles are not brought into use, the **chest sinks,** and all beauty of tone destroyed.

Having condemned the three prevailing systems of breathing - clavicular, costal and diaphragmatic - it will be well to point out peculiarities, defects and disadvantages of each as compared with the **full-chest breathing** method.

CLAVICULAR BREATHING

1. Only the upper part and a portion of the centre of the lungs are brought into use.
2. Correct manipulation of the singing and speaking voice is not possible.
3. With this system nasal breathing in vocalisation, from a practical point of view, is useless.
4. It causes the voice to crack and break on notes in the upper register.
5. By interfering with the management of the correct tension of the vocal cords, it tends to weaken the vocal control.
6. Throat troubles of all descriptions are caused by this system.
7. Greater effort is necessary.
8. Less air is taken into the lungs.
9. The inspirations are more frequent, and the strain is consequently greater.
10. The solidity of tone is impaired, the mode of relaxation interfering with the firm resonance of the air column in the windpipe.
11. Muscles are brought into action which do not belong to the class of breathing muscles at all.
12. It fixes the larynx in one position and makes it stiffen, rendering the tones unmusical.

A few words here may be said in reference to the fixed larynx system advocated by so many singing teachers in these States. This system is the ruin of thousands of voices, being diametrically opposed to the laws of nature - a fact evident to anyone acquainted with the construction of the throat and the actions of the larynx, windpipe and resonance cavities. It is natural for the larynx to rise when high notes are being sung, and to sink for low notes. This has been proved beyong all doubt by such high authorities as Dr G. T Witkowski, Dr Lennox Brown, and others.

COSTAL BREATHING

is an improvement upon clavicular, but still only fills the central and upper parts of the lungs. Control in vocalisation with this system is impossible.

DIAPHRAGMATIC BREATHING

This system is preferable to the preceding two, inasmuch as the parts expanded are more flexible, and so less effort is required; but the amount of air taken in is about the same as with costal breathing, and is, therefore, palpably a faulty method, acting as it does chiefly upon the lower and part of the central lungs. Any method that prevents the thorax being filled in its entirety must be discarded when there is one by which the chest can be wholly filled in a quarter the time required by any other system.

Vocal and Dramatic Studio,
Sydney, London.

Dear Miss Twycross,

You should command success in the profession you have chosen, as you are capable of teaching Voice Production, Full-chest Breathing, &c.

You also possess the artistic, sympathetic temperament, and should be equally successful from the aesthetic standpoint as from the practical.

As it is now the end of the second year you have assisted at my studio, I feel duty bound to send you this special acknowledgement of the valuable services you have rendered.

(Signed) F. MATTHIAS ALEXANDER.

MDLLE. DOLORES

the great singer, eulogised, in a most complimentary letter to Mr Alexander, his method of breathing, a copy of which may be seen at my studio.

FULL-CHEST BREATHING METHOD

I have imparted this full-chest breathing method for some time past, and it has been approved and adopted by leading members of the **medical profession.** Three classes of breathing-gymnastics are imparted, viz.:-

1. Those for the development and control of the muscles used in full inspiration;

2. Exercises which train the muscles used to control the slow relaxation of the lungs in expiration;

3. The exercises which enable the student to take breath quickly through the nostrils.

There is only one way to take a full breath, and that is to cause the whole of the breathing muscles to act together, which can only be accomplished by going through a proper course of

BREATHING GYMNASTICS

suitable to each special case. Every person before being trained has his or her particular way of taking breath, and consequently the breathing-gymnastics which are of value to one person are useless to another.

PROPER MANIPULATION OF THE SINGING VOICE

is not possible with diaphragmatic breathing. Students who learn clavicular, costal or diaphragmatic breathing, and find that breath-taking through the nostrils during vocalisation is not practicable, at once conclude that nasal breathing is a failure in vocal work. This is a mistaken idea, as they would rapidly discover if they understood the art of full-chest breathing.

R. Tait McKenzie, M.D., in a lecture, **"On the Art of Breathing,"** says:- *" The cultivaton of breathing as a fine art is of* ***vital importance*** *to every man, woman and child, but the distance to which it can be carried is a constant surprise to all who see only the results without following the process by which they are obtained. The conditions of modern life make so few calls on* ***great lung capacity*** *that the chest becomes flattened, the lungs cramped, and the shoulders rounded. The muscles of the abdomen become weakened and relaxed by inaction, leaving areas of the lungs practically unused, a fallow for the growth of disease germs. The daily practice of breathing exercises will soon round out the flattened chest and expand the lungs, thus improving health and imparting grace to the carriage. A pair of vigorous lungs well under control are a possession within the reach of every sound man, woman and child who will cultivate them".*

NASAL BREATHING
Full-chest Breathing and Health

The importance of always inhaling through the nostrils must again be emphasised, and cannot be over-estimated, not only in singing and speaking, but in our daily life. Mouth-breathing frequently leads to diseases of the respiratory and vocal organs, nasal growths and catarrh being encouraged by the sensitiveness of the mucous membrane, and inactivity of the nerves and muscles caused by the disuse of the nostrils. The habit of breathing correctly with the -

FULL-CHEST BREATHING METHOD
enabling the student to take in air at all times through the nostrils cannot be acquired too early in life.

Dr Stienbrenner was of the opinion that the habit of superficial breathing was one of the causes of tubercular consumption, and proposed (as **Dr Crighton** and others had done before him) deep breathing as a preventive against consumption.

FAULTS PREVENTED
by the
FULL-CHEST BREATHING METHOD

(Common to Public and Private
Singers and Speakers)

The habit of gasping when inhaling.
Raising the shoulders.
Straining the body out of shape when taking high notes.
Throwing the head back to open the mouth widely.
Falling of the upper chest.
Chest-sinking during singing is a most serious fault. If there is a **solid chest** wall for the windpipe to rest against, the tones will be rounder; but if the chest is allowed to fall in, the windpipe loses its support, and the steadiness and fullness of tone is destroyed.

THROAT TROUBLES
common to 75 per cent of vocal students are invariably caused by the unnatural strain put upon the delicate organs of the throat by
Incorrect Breathing and
Imperfect Production

REMOVE THE STRAIN
from the region of the throat, and the organ will instantly improve, the trouble soon being entirely eradicated.

TO SPEAKERS !

Speakers frequently think that voice-production is unnecessary and quite outside their studies - being of value only to singers. Lisping, defective articulation, nasal tone, & c., are all mechanical faults, all of which may be removed by strengthening the weak parts.

LOSS OF VOICE

Hoarseness and nasal tone in singing or speaking, & c., and most other troubles of their kind, are caused by defective breathing and improper production. Correct production is necessary to enable the speaking voice to develop its full power, and **every singer** should study the art of speaking to perfect the singing voice. The distinct pronunciation of the vowel, together with a perfect articulation of the consonants, should be the aim of every vocalist. Pacchiarotti is quoted as having said, *"He who knows how to breathe and how to pronounce, knows well how to sing"*.

MISS LILIAN TWYCROSS

Vocal Studio :

AUSTRALIAN BUILDINGS,

Corner of Elizabeth Street and Flinders Lane,

MELBOURNE.

Certificated Pupil of

MR. F. M. ALEXANDER,

who introduced the New Methods in Vocalisation and the method of FULL-CHEST BREATHING into Australasia.

Mr. Alexander's Method of Breathing

Eulogised by MDLLE. DOLORES,

The Great Singer.

VARLEY BROS., MELB. & SYD.

DR. ALEXANDER LEEPER

Alexander Leeper (1848 - 1934) was born in Dublin. He was a brilliant classics scholar, completing his education at Trinity College, Dublin, and St. John's College, Oxford. He took up an appointment in 1876 as principal of Trinity College, Melbourne University. He held this position for forty-two years, making a major contribution to the development of collegiate life within the university. As well he was a familiar figure as member of a number of Melbourne educational and cultural organisations, including the Public Library, National Gallery, the Councils of Melbourne Grammar and Melbourne Church of England Girls' Grammar School (leading Melbourne boys and girls schools), the Classical Association and the Shakespeare Society. He was actively involved with church affairs.

It seems unlikely that Dr Leeper had lessons from FM when he taught in Melbourne (1896 - 1900). He did however have lessons in London in 1908, and became a strong supporter of the value of FM's work. Dr Leeper was a member of the Victorian Teachers and Schools Registration Board. This body regulated the standards of teachers who taught at private schools (mainly organised by various religious denominations), either as permanent staff or visiting teachers of specialist subjects. It was a separate body from the State Government Education Department which organised the state-run schools.

In 1908 Dr Leeper was to visit England to attend an Anglican Conference. The Teachers and Schools Registration Board took this opportunity to commission him to investigate and report to the Board on the latest developments in physical culture methods in the United Kingdon and on the Continent. There had been on-going debate in Victoria, and in the whole of Australia, with regard to the merits of the various physical culture systems of the time.

Ths State-run schools did not give as much emphasis to sport and physical culture as did the private schools. There was no formal teacher-training in physical culture. If there was any instruction it was often given to the teacher trainees by army instructors. Once out teaching, they would give their pupils mainly marching drills, plus a few other exercises of an elementary nature.

A number of the private schools regarded sport and physical culture as an integral part of the school curriculum. Some games were played as inter-school sports, particlulary well organised amongst the boys' schools, while in the girls' schools certain types of callisthenic exercises, and later the Swedish

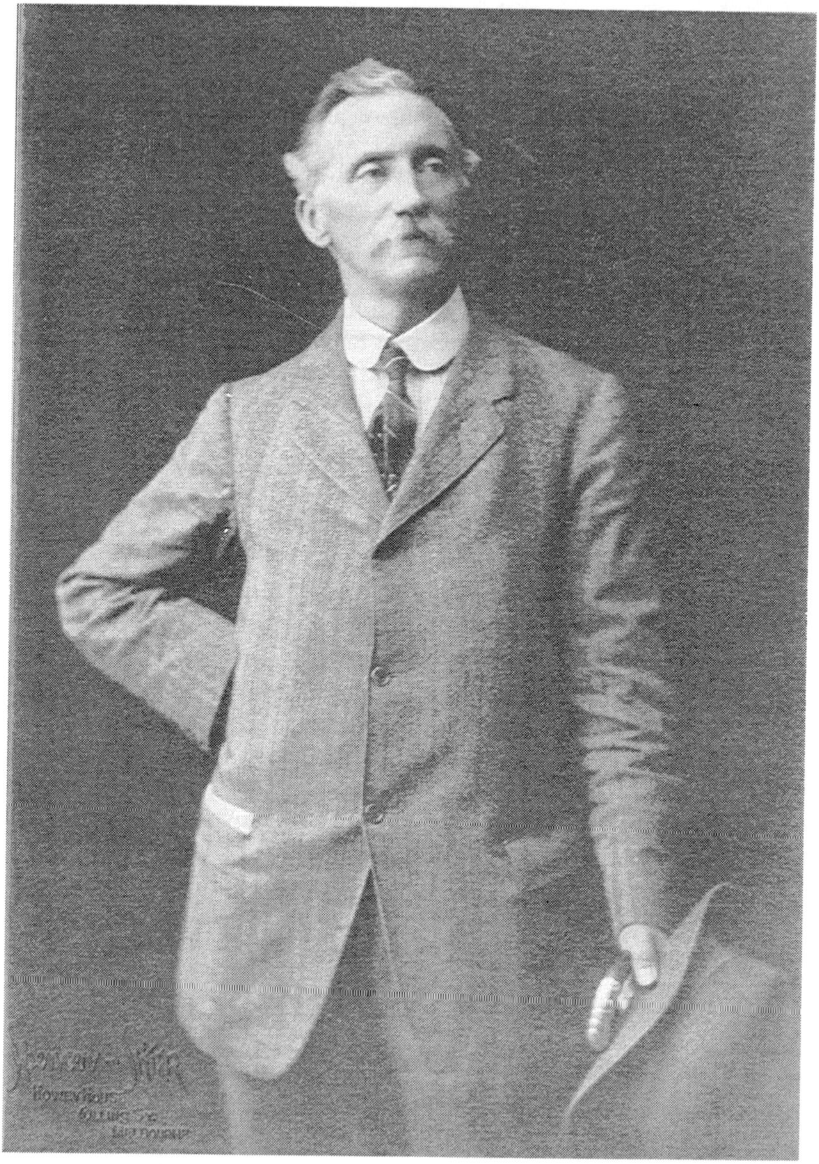

Dr. Alexander Leeper
(Courtesy of Trinity College, Melbourne University)

drills, became part of the curriculum. There was interest in and attention given to what was happening in England with regard to games and physical culture, so it is not surprising that in 1908 when the Victorian Teachers and Schools Registration Board was deciding on standards for sport/physical culture teachers, and the type of training they should have, a Report on the whole subject should be commissioned.

The Report on Physical Culture in the United Kingdon and the Continent of Europe by Dr Leeper was presented to the Victorian Teachers and Schools Registration Board in March 1909. It is of particular interest to Alexander teachers, given its references to Dr Leeper's experience in England in relation to FM's work. Major portions of this Report are now quoted:

" *When I was leaving on a visit to England last year, I was requested by the Board to examine and report upon the latest developments of physical culture in the United Kingdom and on the Continent of Europe. The subject is a large one, and for its proper study would have demanded far more time and attention than it was possible for me to devote to it. More than this, one really needs to have passed through a complete course of physical training oneself in order to be in a position to pronounce with any confidence on the relative merits or defects of the various systems favoured by the authorites on education. Circumstances compelled me to confine my examination of the subject, such as it was, wholly to England, and only one branch of physical culture, viz., breathing exercises and voice production, was I able to make a subject of special study....It seems to be recognised in England that what has been called a `health conscience' is a necessary part of the equipment of a good teacher, and that the teacher cannot, in justice to his class and to the State, regard the health and bodily development of his scholars as matters lying outside his department. Everywhere I noticed a great quickening of interest in the physical side of education. I found, however, a strong conflict of opinion upon the relative values of the various systems in vogue. As to this point, Sir Robert Morant, the Permanent Secretary of the Board of Education, in a letter which he wrote to me last September, said:*

'There is acute diversity of views in England as to physical exercises, as in every other portion of the educational field. We are certainly not stagnant here, but we are too fertile of new notions'.

" *The Swedish exercises are, perhaps, the most generally favoured, especially in girls' schools and in the case of at least one great public school, the physical culture master was sent to Stockholm to go through the whole course of the exercises in one of the Government gymnasiums in order that he might be qualified to teach Ling's system in its entirety on his return; but, while the Swedish system has its many ardent supporters, it has been of late the object also of much severe criticism by experts. The respiratory move-*

ments, for example, which form so marked a feature of the system, are emphatically condemned by some well-recognised experts in voice production and elocution....

" *This brings me to that particular branch of physical culture to which I gave most attention during my visit to England, and which, I believe, is coming to be recognised alike by doctors, singing teachers, and elocutionists as a prime necessity in physical training. I mean breathing exercises and correct voice production. The fundamental importance of these is strongly forcing itself on the attention of the whole teaching profession in England. Training in breathing and in voice production has been made an essential part of the curriculum of every teacher under the Board of Education. In the latest syllabus of physical exercises issued by the Board of Education, it is insisted that deep-breathing exercises should form part of the daily training of every scholar, and efforts are to be made to teach, even in the infant school, the correct method of nasal-respiration. I wonder in how many secondary schools of Victoria is any attempt of the kind made. Yet it seems particularly desirable that voice training should be included in the ordinary curriculum of Australian schools; for it is vain to deny that an unpleasant drawl and a want of a clear distinction between the vowel sounds are beginning to be noticed abroad as characteristic of Australian pronunciation, and they are not always absent from the speech of our educated folk. We have the disagreeable American twang before us as awful warning what the neglect of proper articuation may lead to.*

" *I do not believe that our defect is due to climatic influences or to any other unavoidable local condition. It is simply a matter of training. I could name a school in Melbourne where the boys' articulation is perfect, and their vowel sounds are produced as distinctly and euphoniously as any could desire. This is due, I believe, wholly to the fact that they are all, from the beginning, carefully taught breathing, voice production, and singing. What can be done in one school might be done in all. In this department, also, just as in the case of gymnastics, there are many competing systems, and in England, at any rate, no kind of finality has as yet been reached. I have given a good deal of attenion to some of the various methods, and have formed a definite opinion as to which is the best of those that came under my observation. I should without hesitation, give the first place to the system associated with the name of Mr F. Matthias Alexander, who it will interest the Board to know, is a Victorian by birth and education.* (Ed. Tasmanian by birth.) *He taught in Melbourne for some years. He has now settled in London, and has further developed, and, as he thinks, perfected his method of what he calls respiratory re-education. He has secured very remarkable results. It would take too long and in any case it would be difficult merely by oral explanation to make clear to the Board the rationale of his method. More than that, I am inclined to think that it is not possible to give a really satisfactory and scientific elucidation and that there is some element of chance in the discoveries on which he has lighted. The main features which seem to distinguish it from rival systems are :-*

1. The inflation of the lungs with the maximum air and the minimum of exertion;
2. the use of pose rather than of muscular effort to assist the breathing;
3. the gaining of a perfect control over the breath, so that the process of inhaling, whether in reading, speaking, reciting, or singing is absolutely imperceptible.

" The results are most striking. It is no exaggeration to say that most of the leaders of the dramatic profession in London (and what better judges could possibly be found?) are enthusiastic believers in the efficacy of his system, and many of them have placed themselves under him for tuition. One of his pupils, it may be mentioned, is Miss Lily Brayton, who will soon be performing to Australian audiences, and whose vocalization is, I believe, considered as simply faultless. Not only did I take a course of lessons, myself, but I went to the trouble of making personal acquaintance with some of the members of the dramatic profession who had been in Mr Alexander's hands. Mr and Mrs H. B. Irving bore strong testimony to the astonishing efficacy of his treatment. Mr Irving said to me, 'I cannot exaggerate the value of his method. He has simply made a new man of me.' Mr Beerbohm Tree, whose stage voice is the envy of his profession, seemed to be no less appreciative. I have seen letters from other leaders of the profession, testifying in the warmest terms to Mr Alexander's powers. I also wrote to several specialists in London, who have been sending patients to Mr Alexander for the cure of defects of speech, throat vocalization, and chest weakness. They one and all speak of the results as entirely satisfactory. For example, Dr Scanes Spicer, an eminent throat specialist and lecturer on diseases of the throat in London University, wrote to me :-

" 'The results, not only in the production of the voice, but also in the deportment, appearance, and general health surpass anything that I have hitherto met with. Among the chief points which distinguish his practice from that of other physical educators are:

1. The absolute avoidance of physical strain, so conserving the available energy of the body;
2. the thorough emptying of the chest on expiration in such a way as to let the respiratory act be to some extent an elastic recoil;
3. the prevention of undue suction of the mucous membrane of the throat by insisting on no gasping or sniffing;

4. the better position of the thoracic and abdominal viscera, and the holding of the weight of the body to the best mechanical advantage'.

" The complete scientific explanation of the subject is not yet possible; but the results are in an unusual degree beneficial, and worthy of the attention of all medical and educational authorities. Dr Jakins, of Harley-street, another well-known specialist writes :-

'I have sent a number of patients to Mr Alexander. I am of the opinion that the principles of his method are far in advance of any other physical or breathing culture known to me'.

" Sir Alfred Fripp, surgeon-in-ordinary to the King wrote :- 'I have certainly been much impressed with the good results I have seen accomplished by Mr Alexander's methods.'

" Dr Bruce Porter of 6 Grosvenor-street, also bears testimony to the great value of Mr Alexander's principles and methods. Mr Alexander's brother is now carrying on his system of training in Melbourne. I am informed by Dr Smyth, of the Training College, that last winter Mr Alexander gave the State school teachers a course of lessons in breathing exercises, with which Dr Smyth told me he was most favorably impressed. I have asked Mr Alexander whether he would be willing to give a short demonstration of his brother's method some day to the Registration Board, and he said he would be very glad to do so, and to answer any questions that members might like to ask.

" No apparatus of any kind is required, and, as far as the exercises themselves are concerned, they are of a very simple character, and easily performed.

" As the outcome of what I have seen and heard during my trip to England, I venture, with all the diffidence becoming one who is conscious that he is in no sense an expert, and who claims to be, as an observer, fitted with nothing more than average intelligence, to make the following suggestions to the Board :

1. That, wherever local conditions allow, swimming be insisted upon as one of the first essentials of education, whether for boys or girls.
2. That the systematic records of the physical condition of the pupils be periodically collected and reserved in all schools.
3. That compulsory medical inspection of all schools form part of the Board's programme.
4. That the Registration Board take into consideration the question whether it would not be wise to seek for the appointment of a Royal Commission to report upon physical culture for schools.
5. That a more prominent place be given in our schools to correct breathing

and voice production, and that good vocalization be recognised as one of the best tests of a sound and well co-ordinated physique.
6. That what is known as the Alexander method of the re-education of the respiratory organs is deserving of the Board's special attention.
8th March, 1909".

Though the Dr Leeper Report was circulated to schools for comment, certainly the sections relating to the Alexander work were not acted upon. This is not surprising. AR Alexander left Melbourne for England in 1911. Miss Twycross, a former assistant to FM, was mainly a teacher of singing, though she also possessed a physical culture qualification. However, there were in Melbourne several schools of Physical Culture, or Gymnasiums, whose instructors were often used as visiting specialists; and also some school staff had travelled overseas for specialist training in various branches of physical culture. Given the presence in Melbourne of these two strong physical culture strands, the now small and tenuous foothold of the Alexander work was not likely to attract major attention. Had FM stayed in Melbourne the strong clientele he had built up between 1896 - 1900 may have given a solid enough base which would have convinced the 1909 Schools and Teachers Registration Board to weigh more deeply the merit of Alexander's work in comparison with the claims of the other physical culture systems of that time.

It is interesting to note that in the Dr Leeper Report the term physical culture, for him, includes consideration of breathing and voice production. This broad interpretation of the term physical culture seems not to have been taken up by others. During the next few years, as governments became more interested in the fitness of youth, their concern , especially for boys, was that there be adequate preparation of cadets by a schedule of exercises and drills, fully laid out in prescribed manuals.

Though the recommendation in the Leeper Report on the merits of Alexander's work was not taken up by the Board, Dr Leeper himself did have further contact with FM, and in the archival collection of his papers there are several articles relating to physical health and in particular to Alexander's work. Dr Leeper's interests were wide and his contacts far-reaching. The extracts on physical health come from both British and Australian newspapers.

The Onlooker, a British paper, printed two considerations of FM's book, Man's Supreme Inheritance, under the heading Health and Hygiene. The first article was on October 22nd, 1910 with a sub-heading, A Revolutionary Thesis, and it concluded as follows:

" *In place, therefore, of physical culture or purely psychic therapeutics as a safeguard against the deterioration engendered by an artificial existence, Mr Alexander's theory indicates a system of what I can only describe as psycho-physiological treatment, whereby the conscious intellect or will power may be trained to control the sub-conscious functions of mind and body. It is, indeed, a big proposition. But the application of this theory to practice is so fascinating and suggestive that I hope to have an opportunity of referring to it again".*

The second article, October 29th, 1910, had as sub-heading, " A Plea for Re-education". The following are two extracts from this article:

" *Physical deterioration is, in the minds of the vast majority of people, associated with enfeebled muscular devlopment. It is, of course, not necessarily anything of the kind. A man, for example, may - often is - deteriorate in such vital functions as the proper equilibrium of the body, or in the vital functions of the respiratory system, and still be muscularly a model to delight a sculptor's eyes. The whole of the fallacy of what is known as the 'physical culture' vogue lies in attaching undue consideration to the development of certain groups of visible muscles. Physical culture is, in fact, in ninety-nine cases out of a hundred, an attempt to correct misapprehended defects by irrational methods...Infinitely more important towards the attainment of physical fitness than any muscular development is the correction of those deep-seated defects, such as faulty equilibrium in the habitual pose (as was illustrated by photographs in our issue last week) and wrong methods of breathing - defects due in the first place to the artificiality of the conditions of civilised life, but unfortunately confirmed and inculcated by educational methods, ignorant or reckless of the most elementary knowledge of the mechanism of the body. These bedrock defects, in their turn, affect all the vital organs which we have come to regard as exercising their functions subconsciously - for example, the lungs, the heart, and the digestive apparatus.*

" *It is against these more deep-seated and unrecognised defects that Mr Alexander directs his efforts, and his methods have, in practice, been endorsed by the more enlightened and liberal section of medical opinion".*

The subject of Deep Breathing, a definition of it, whether it should be taught (especially in schools) and how it should be taught were topics of at times quite heated debate. Copies in the Leeper archives of letters to the editor in the British paper, Pall Mall Gazette, show divided opinion about the subject. One letter includes a suggestion to other letter writers that they should read Mr Alexander's publications on the subject. The correspondence on the issue was eventually brought to a close by the Pall Mall Gazette Editor.

In 1919 FM wrote to Dr Leeper from New York sending him *"some matter which I think will interest you"*. This included publicity material about

Man's Supreme Inheritance and copies of appreciation of the book by various prominent people, including American educator and philosopher John Dewey. In 1924 FM wrote to Dr Leeper and included a complimentary copy of his book 'Constructive Conscious Control of the Individual'.

Dr Leeper's life spanned a period of great change. He was passionate about some things and interested in many others. Some of his enthusiasms - such as wanting to establish a collegiate university residence for women, in which he succeeded - were innovative and ahead of his times. Dr Leeper's opinions sometimes caused difficulties, but his overall influence in the community was widespread and benefited the educational and cultural life of Melbourne. Of the four children from his first marriage, the two sons both settled in England and rose to prominence in the British Foreign Office. Sir Reginald Leeper (1888 - 1968) was a diplomat and the 'architect' of the British Council. Had there been a stronger Alexander 'base' in Victoria during Dr Alexander Leeper's life, no doubt he would have given the Alexander method stronger encouragement and support during the years of protracted debate about physical culture and its role in education.

SYDNEY

When FM decided to move from Melbourne to Sydney in early 1900, change was in the air. The six colonies were on the brink of Federation. Much hard work had been done over a number of years to bring this about. Conventions had been held, Constitutions drafted, and the opinion of the people gathered via referenda. There was a clear movement towards the uniting of the separate colonies. The Southern Baptist newspaper, February 16th, 1899, expressed this sentiment as follows, *"Federation appears to be nearer to-day than ever before. We congratulate the Premiers of the several colonies upon the solution of the huge difficulties which were presented for their discussion. Our hope is that the new century, when its gates shall open, will find a new nation in existence, bearing the euphonious name of Australia".*

On January 1st, 1901, Federation became a reality and the Commonwealth of Australia was born. The capital of the Commonwealth was yet to be decided, and temporary headquarters were in Melbourne. After much soul-searching and delay (including Australia's involvement in World War I) a site was finally chosen, and an architect-designed city established. Canberra, the new capital for the Federal Parliament of Australia, was opened in 1927 with much pomp and ceremony.

Sydney was the oldest and dominant city of the colonies until the 1850's, when Victoria, with its tremendous gold boom became the richer colony, and the capital Melbourne usurped Sydney's position. During the turbulence of the 1890's the financial crashes, the collapse of the real estate boom etc. hit Victoria hardest. In 1901, at the time of federation, both Sydney and Melbourne had populations of half a million. In the ensuing years, Sydney, which recovered from the depression more quickly than Melbourne, again became the biggest city.

The natural resources of Sydney include one of the world's most beautiful harbours. To leave or approach Sydney by ship, through the heads, is unquestionably to experience Nature in its full grandeur. The city of Sydney itself has many fine buildings around the foreshore. The theatre tradition was a strong one and, as in Melbourne, there were a number of theatres, whose place in Sydney's cultural life was well established. When FM settled there in early 1900 there would have been ample scope for him to establish himself both as reciter and teacher.

Sydney was to be FM's home for four years. His first aim was to establish himself as a vocal art teacher, and to this end he also gave recitals which would bring him attention not only as a reciter, but also as someone who had particular knowledge to impart about the Human Voice. His advertisements to publicize his Vocal Studio were sometimes large and explanatory.

The following appeared in the Sydney Morning Herald on March 17th, 1900. (All following advertisements quoted, unless otherwise specified are from the Sydney Morning Herald.)

"

THE HUMAN VOICE

Cultivated and Developed for

SPEAKING and SINGING
by
THE NEW METHODS

at Mr F. M. ALEXANDER'S VOCAL STUDIO
Equitable-buildings, George-street, Sydney,

as imparted by him during the PAST 4 YEARS in MELBOURNE

He is preparted to receive Students for the Study of
NATURAL ELOCUTION CULTIVATION
and
DRAMATIC TRAINING
of the SPEAKING and SINGING VOICE
PROPER MANIPULATION and PRODUCTION.
Cure Throat Troubles (Clergyman's Sore Throat),
Breaks, Faulty Notes (Singing and Speaking Voice).

FULL CHEST BREATHING
A new and improved method, which governs the production and gives thorough control for the voice.
BREATHING GYMNASTICS
for the development of the human chest.
STUTTERING etc.,
and all Vocal Impediments removed by New and Natural Methods

TREATISE OF VOCAL CULTURE,
giving particulars regarding the new methods, breathing, production, manipulations, and the proper course of study to pursue, may be obtained, FREE OF CHARGE, at the Studio, or will be posted on receipt of stamp".

To conclude the advertisement FM listed the names of nineteen well-known Melbournians who had given him testimonials. The originals of these were available at FM's studios for perusal.

By September FM had settled in and was ready to make his first major Sydney stage appearance. The recital was at the Centenary Hall on September 1st. FM's associate artists included Mr Robert Young and Miss Edith Tasca-Page. His recitations included some old favorties, 'The Clock Mystery' and scenes from Shakespeare and Dickens. The recital advertisement also included reference to FM's teaching work. The whole performance was much appreciated by the audience and the critics were generous with praise.

Encouraged by this success, a second entertainment was announced for September 15th. Now the heading was, "ALEXANDER -YOUNG - PAGE ENTERTAINMENTS".
The advertisement for this performance continued as follows,

REFINED MIRTH
DELIGHTFUL MUSIC,
WIT and HUMOUR.
INTELLECTUAL ENTERTAINMENT.
Second appearance of
Mr F. M. ALEXANDER
Mr ROBERT YOUNG
Miss EDITH TASCA-PAGE,
who were received by a large audience on the success of their first appearance with
UNBOUNDED ENTHUSIASM".

There was then detail about each performer's items and after the name of Mr Robert Young there was, in brackets, "(a la Corney Grain and George Grossmith.)" Below the large recital advertisement were two small advertisements for FM's teaching at the Equitable Building, George Street Sydney.

In 1901 the tenants on the fifth floor of the Equitable Building, studios 5 - 6, were listed as FM Alexander, Signor Rossi, Professor of Music, R. F. Young and Miss Edith Tasca-Page. On January 12th, 1901 FM advertised his teaching methods, but in addition there is a larger advertisement headed, "The Merchant of Venice". Then follows, *"Mr F. M. Alexander will stage the "Merchant of Venice" early this year, interpreting Shylock himself, and will receive applications from those desirous of appearing in the production".*

A passion for Shakespeare's plays had been and was to remain part of FM's life. From childhood he had delighted in the study of the Bard's works. Now that he was well-established in Sydney here was the opportunity to mount his own production, casting his own pupils. What better way to demonstrate the efficacy of his teaching methods?

The advertisements in the Sydney Morning Herald of February 9th, 16th and 23rd all carry information about FM's dual activities as teacher and producer of The Merchant of Venice. It is interesting to note that one of FM's co-tenants, R. F. Young, put a large advertisement in the Sydney Morning Herald of February 16th and 23rd announcing his School of Physical Culture, and that he taught the Sandow System. By mid 1901 FM had prepared his Shakespearean class for public performance.

The Theatre Royal, Sydney, was the venue for The Merchant of Venice, directed by FM Alexander, who also played Shylock; other cast included Edith Tasca-Page as Portia and a number of ladies and gentlemen selected from FM's Shakespearean class. There were three performances, June 27th, 28th and 29th. They were under the patronage of, and on one occasion in the presence of, His Excellency, the Lieutenant-Govenor, Sir F. M. Darley, G.C.M.G. On July 6th the Sydney Morning Herald carried a large advertisement beginning with several lines of gracious thanks from FM to the people of Sydney for the support they gave him for the Merchant of Venice production. Then follows the outline of an ambitious project to mount several more Shakespeare plays, the casts to be chosen from "Mr Alexander's Shakespearean Society" and that he will form a professional company next year. Underneath this are extensive quotes from several of the enthusiastic reviews of the recent Merchant of Venice performances.

Nineteen hundred and two promised to be a big year for FM. On January 18th he announced that the first term at the Sydney Dramatic and Operatic Conservatorium would begin on February 17th and that copies of the prospectus were available from the secretary. A further advertisement appeared on January 25th as follows:

"SYDNEY DRAMATIC AND OPERATIC CONSERVATORIUM,
84 Hunter street, near Phillip street.
Under the patronage of
His Excellency the Lieutenant-Governor, Sir F. M. Darley, G.C.M.G.
Director, Mr F. M. ALEXANDER

The success which has attended Mr F. M. Alexander's Shakespearean production in Sydney has proved so gratifying that he has decided to establish a Dramatic and Operatic Conservatorium. The Director has engaged a competent staff of Professional Assistants, and Dramatic and Operatic (classical) Performances will be arranged at intervals at a Sydney Theatre, in which the whole of the characters will be interpreted by Students of the Conservatorium. A special feature in the course of study will be the famous

DELSARTE SYSTEM

as applied to dramatic expression, deportment, gestures, and vocalisation. It will be generally admitted that this system is of the greatest educational and artistic value, for it is an aesthetic science with the same precision as mathematical science. Its proper application gives perfection to vocalisation, poetry of gesture, grace and distinction in motion, and the combined action of the physical and spiritual.

TO OPERATIC AND SINGING STUDENTS

The Director has great pleasure in announcing that he has especially engaged the well-known Conductor and Teacher of Singing

HERR SLAPOFFSKI

in connection with the Operatic Course at the Conservatorium. NOTE.- The course of study at the Conservatorium has been so arranged that it will prove as valuable to the ORDINARY STUDENT of SINGING and SPEAKING as to the stage aspirant.

The following are Dramatic Studies which will be rehearsed for production: "Much Ado About Nothing", "Othello", "Twelfth Night", "School for Scandal", and "Pygmalion and Galatea." First term begins Feb. 17th. All communications should be addressed to the Secretary, Sydney Dramatic and Operatic Conservatorium, 84 Hunter street".

Two new names feature prominently here with FM for the first time. They are Delsarte, the "famous DELSARTE SYSTEM" and Herr Slapoffski.

Francois Delsarte (1811 - 1871) was a French actor who achieved fame for the methods he developed of acting, mime, gesture and breathing. He was paid the highest tributes in France for his teaching. Knowledge of his methods spread, particularly in America, where his work achieved great popularity in the latter part of the nineteenth century. Though Delsarte never visited this country, supporters of his work brought it to the attention of the public. For the last ten years of his life, Delsarte was in ill health, and he died in relative obscurity. He did not publish very much of his work but knowledge of it has been kept alive by the writings of others, though some of the accuracy of this has been questioned.

One of the best books about Delsarte and his method is called 'Every Little Movement' by Ted Shawn. Delsarte himself is quoted, *"Gesture is more than speech. It is not what we say that persuades, but the manner of saying it. Speech is inferior to gesture because it corresponds to the phenomena of mind. Gesture is the agent of the heart, the persuasive agent".*

During a lecture tour in America Delsarte's daughter, *"emphasized that her father never taught gymnastics, but lectured on a science of expression which he had evolved".*

During the 1890's, " *Besides the large number of `Delsarte' books which related to gymnastics, physical culture, and expressive gesture - there was an equally large number of books put out for the use of the orator, the elocutionist, the reader of recitations*".

Re Delsarte's pupils, his "*classes were attended by actors, opera singers, statesmen, lawyers, great preachers from pulpits - all who used voice with gesture; but that not a single dancer, so far as we have been able to discover, attended his classes or lectures*".

There is reference to an article published in 1897 titled 'Delsarte and His Contribution to Physical Education' by Mrs.Anna P.Tucker. Ted Shawn writes, "*In this article, Mrs.Tucker deplores the distortions of the true science of Delsarte, but maintains that using the science with deep understanding, and correctly, is the basis of the finest possible system of physical education. She makes comparisons between the mechanical gymnastics, the athletic-sport training program (prevalent today as it was then) and the ideal goals, aims and ends of a real physical education - and based on her own teaching, shows why this science does and can produce the finest possible results. The facts and the arguments in this article are as valid today as they were in 1887, and I wish this could be read by all teachers of physical education, as well as by teachers of dance in physical education departments.*"

Much of the work published about Delsarte is derivative. One can only speculate at present as to how FM came across Delsarte's work here in Australia. It could have been by reading, it could have been by coming in contact with actors from abroad who came to Australia to perform or teach and who had knowledge of Delsarte's methods. However FM came upon his work, it obviously struck a chord in him and for a time he enthusiastically espoused the Delsarte system.

The professional association between FM and Herr Slapoffski seems to have been short-term. Slapoffski was to take the operatic classes for FM's Sydney Dramatic and Operatic Conservatorium, announced to commence in February 1902. Herr Gustave Slapoffski (1862 - 1951) had a distinguished career as a musician. He was born in London, his father was a Russian-born musician, his mother an Australian, born in Sydney. As a youngster Slapoffski was a very talented violinist, who eventually became leader of the Carl Rosa Opera Company orchestra and later chief conductor. In 1900 Slapoffski was engaged as musical director for an opera season in Australia. Slapoffski's wife, a highly respected singer, was to be a soloist with the company.

From then on Australia became home for the Slapoffskis. They were deeply involved with many aspects of Australian musical life, performing, teaching etc. Until about 1930 they were Sydney-based, then they moved to Melbourne and continued an active musical life for many years.

Advertisements for FM's Sydney Dramatic and Operatic Conservatorium appeared regularly for a short time in 1902, then ceased. Such an ambitious project appears not to have been possible. Later in the year FM resumed the advertising of his vocal teaching at his Sydney studio. As well an advertisement for March 8th, 1902 announced,

"NEW DRAMATIC COMPANY

Four Ladies and Six Gentlemen required for
MR. F. MATTHIAS ALEXANDER'S
NO. 2 TOURING COMPANY

Lady and Gentleman (with professional experience) to play leading parts.

Applications by letter only are invited from Professional and Amateur Dramatic Artists for other characters.
Write the Stage Manager, 84 Hunter-street, Sydney".

Obviously FM was still combining his theatre work and teaching.

The year 1903 was to see FM changing the direction of his work from the more specific vocal and breathing area to the all-embracing field of general health. An advertisement for January 24th, 1903 reads,

"POST NASAL GROWTHS

THROAT and CHEST TROUBLES,
STUTTERING and STAMMERING,
CULTIVATION SPEAKING and SINGING VOICE,
FULL-CHEST BREATHING METHOD.

Treatise on the above forwarded free on application to Secretary,

MR. F. M. ALEXANDER'S Vocal Studio,
Tattersall's-chambers, corner
Hunter and Castlereagh Streets".

The February advertisements include reference to a "Eulogistic Letter received from Mdlle. Dolores" endorsing FM's methods. She was a visiting singer, to whom FM had apparently sent material about his methods, of which she approved. Reference is still made by FM to teaching the "FAMOUS DELSARTE SYSTEM".

In December 1903 FM Alexander made very public the major shift in his work to that of an overall concept of health. An advertisement of December 5th, 1903 announced,

"A N E W B O O K A N E W B O O K
A N E W B O O K A N E W B O O K

ON
NEW
METHODS

by F. M A T T H I A S A L E X A N D E R
(who has imparted his NEW METHOD for ten years in Australasia)

A Book on a subject of VITAL IMPORTANCE and UNIVERSAL INTEREST - THE ART OF BREATHING,and embodying the details of a

PERFECT BREATHING METHOD
PERFECT BREATHING METHOD

(securing the maximum of expansion and contraction with the minimum of effort), as imparted in connection with:

1. - THE TREATMENT OF DISEASE

PREVENTION or CURE of Throat , Lung (Consumption, etc.), CHEST, HEART, NERVE, LIVER and STOMACH (Indigestion etc.) DISORDERS, POST-NASAL (ADENOID) GROWTHS, the AFTER-EFFECTS OF PLEURISY, and IMPEDIMENT OF SPEECH.

2.- THE CULTIVATION AND DEVELOPMENT OF THE HUMAN VOICE
(Perfect Art in Singing and Speaking).

3. - PHYSICAL CULTURE AND BODY BUILDING
(a perfect system of Physical Development, having a correct and natural primary movement for each exercise).

AN IMPORTANT FACT

In connection with the diseases enumerated under heading No. 1, the author has treated patients recommended by Dr.Brady, Dr.W.J.Stewart McKay, Dr.Reginald Bowman, and Dr.Hogg, of Sydney; and Dr.Kenny, Dr.Stawell, Dr.Charles Bage, and Dr.D.S.MacColl, of Melbourne; and has received most eulogistic letters concerning his methods from Mdlle. Dolores, Dr.Charles Bage, Professor Harrison Moore (Melb.University), J.C.Williamson, Esq., Rev.Prior Kelly, Dr.D.S.MacColl, E.W.Rathbone, Esq., (London Art Critic), Miss Mabel Ward (Contralto Vocalist), Rev.E.Handel Jones, Robert Brough, Esq., Professor Whitely (Baptist Theological College), Arthur Robinson, Esq., (Solicitor), H.C.Geoghegan, Esq., (Barrister), Frederic Villiers, Esq., D.C.Rees, Esq., (Lands Titles Office, Melb.).

OPINIONS

Dr.CHARLES BAGE writes, "*After a course of lessons from you I am fully convinced that your confidence in the correctness of your methods is abundantly justified.*"

Dr.D.S.MacCOLL writes, "*I am confident that your methods are excellent. The bearer, Rev. ....., is suffering with a throat affliction; I am confident you can help him.*"

PRACTICAL VALUE OF THE BOOK

This Book will prove of great value and practical assistance to

PARENTS,

enabling them to impart to THEIR CHILDREN a perfect breathing method, which will tend to prevent PULMONARY DISEASES, POST-NASAL (ADENOID) GROWTHS, and other defects tending to cause nasal stenosis.

Dr. SEARES SPICER,
Surgeon, Throat Department, St.Mary's Hospital, London, when advocating the study and practice of breathing as a preventative of ADENOID growths, etc. said: "*As a matter of fact the MANNER OF BREATHING of every child, just as much as its food and clothing, housing and air, exercise, bathing and education, requires constant and unremitting attention from the moment of birth*".

A Practical and Valuable Book for
VOCAL STUDENTS, TEACHERS, LAYMEN, AND EXPERTS, who desire to secure the marvellous benefits to be derived from a perfect breathing method in all VOCAL EFFORT, or in the TREATMENT of THE DISEASES already enumerated.

SPECIAL SETS OF BREATHING EXERCISES
SPECIAL SETS OF NASAL AND BREATHING EXERCISES
SPECIAL SETS OF PHYSICAL EXERCISES

These exercises are most minutely described, and the ILLUSTRATIONS in connection with them will be taken from photographs of the author in the act of the demonstration of his methods. The author feels justified in stating that the Breathing Exercises are the MOST PRACTICAL and COMPLETE that have so far been published.

NOTE

A pamphlet containing full and detailed particulars of the CONTENTS OF THE BOOK will be forwarded to any address on receipt of stamp.

PARTICULARS OF PUBLICATION.

This Book will NOT be "on sale" in the ordinary way, as only sufficient copies will be published to supply the orders received. The book will be delivered as early as possible in the coming year,1904. Address order to Mr.F.Matthias Alexander, Royal-chambers, corner of Hunter and Castlereagh Streets, Sydney, where his methods are imparted. Interviews should be arranged by letter".

The book was entitled, 'Breathing, Vocalisation and Physical Culture', and cost ten shillings and sixpence including delivery.

Following this long advertisement, the Daily Telegraph of December 12th, 1903 carried an article by FM titled, ' The Prevention and Cure of Consumption' FM had received particular encouragement and support from Dr.W.J.Stewart McKay to have this article published. It deals with breathing, what faulty breathing does to the body, and how improvement of breathing influences body function. (The full text of this article by FM and other articles he wrote during his many years of teaching will be published in book form in England in 1995.)

Clients, Contacts, and a Colleague

Clients

Following the Melbourne pattern, FM had a cross-section of students, including politicians, clergy, lawyers and doctors. Two prominent people who encouraged FM were Judge Charles Murray and Dr. W. J. Stewart McKay.

Judge Charles Murray (1842-1923) was born in London and the family came to Australia in 1852. He attended school in Sydney then went on to Sydney University where he showed high scholastic ability. He was called to the Bar in 1867 and in 1878 was appointed a Judge of the District Court, continuing in this job until ill-health forced his retirement in 1916.

Dr William John Stewart McKay (1866-1948) was born and educated in Sydney, graduating in medicine from Sydney University in 1891. He went to England, and following a short stay as resident medical officer at the Soho Hospital for Women, moved to Birmingham to work as assistant to Lawson Tait, a surgeon of world wide fame. After returning to Sydney Dr. McKay began private practice and in 1895 joined the staff of the Lewisham Hospital, with which he was to be associated for over thirty years. Dr. McKay had a broad scientific outlook on many subjects, including knowledge of animals. His writings covered such topics as medical history, surgery, biography, comparative anatomy and racehorses. Dr. McKay's interest in horses was both technical (Evolution of the Endurance, Speed and Staying Power of the Racehorse, two editions, 1933 and 1937) and for pleasure, another interest being the theatre. Dr. McKay had heard from colleagues in Melbourne about the merit of FM's work. So when FM came to live in Sydney in 1900, Dr.McKay was curious to find out just how good FM's work was. He was not disappointed, and gave FM strong support. When FM went to London in 1904, armed with letters of reference, those from Dr.McKay would have carried considerable weight.

Contacts

Robert Brough, one of Australia's great actor-managers, gave FM an encouraging letter of commendation about his recitations fairly early in FM's career. Robert Brough and his wife, who first came to Australia in 1885 for a Gilbert and Sullivan season, were both from the D'Oyly Carte Opera Company in London. In 1886 the Brough-Boucicault Company was formed and began performances in Sydney. For ten years this company was one of the mainstays of Australian theatre. Robert Brough then formed his own company, which toured in Australia and overseas. Brough worked abroad for a number of years before returning to Australia. He died in Sydney in 1906.

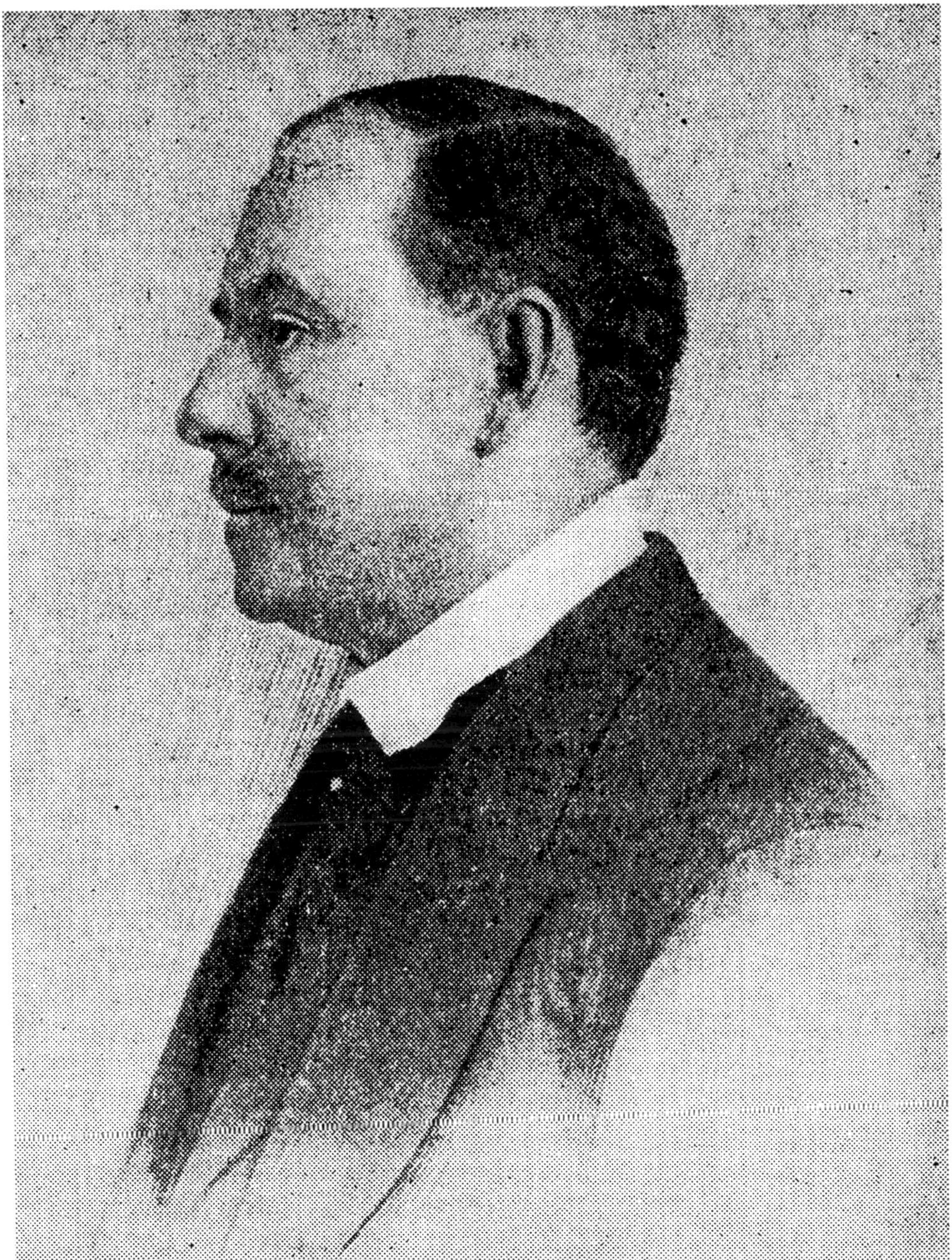

Dr. J W S McKay (copyright © the Medical Journal of Australia 1967; II:931. Reprinted with permission.)
(Courtesy of La Trobe Collection, State Library of Victoria)

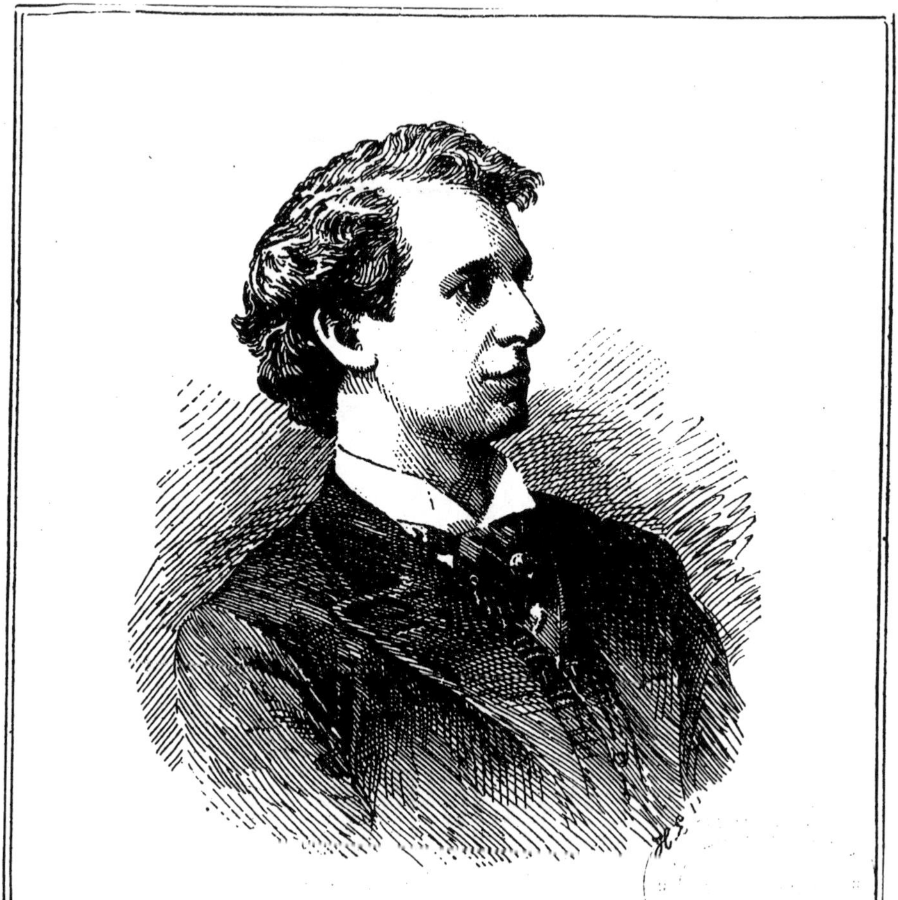

MR. WALTER BENTLEY, TRAGEDIAN.—FROM A PHOTOGRAPH BY THE VANDYCK STUDIO.

Walter Bentley (Courtesy of La Trobe Collection, State Library of Victoria)

The eulogistic letter about FM's methods from the French soprano, Antonia Dolores, was one which FM prominently displayed in some of his advertisements. Mdlle. Dolores had made her Australian debut in 1895 under her original name Antoinette Trebelli. She was to tour Australia with great success a number of times, the last visit being in 1920.

Reference has already been made to the strong impression the acting of Walter Bentley made on FM in Melbourne in the early 1890's and which resulted in FM writing a tragic poem, 'The Dream of Matthias the Burgomaster', inspired by Bentley's performance in the play, 'The Bells'. The paths of Walter Bentley and FM Alexander were to cross a number of times, and the influence of the older actor cannot be doubted.

Walter Bentley (1849-1927) was born and educated in Edinburgh, Scotland. His course was set for the ministry, but it was a path with which he did not agree, and he ran away to sea. This soon brought him to Australia; he jumped ship in Sydney in 1867, and not long after became a rouseabout on a cattle station in Queensland. In 1871 Bentley went to New Zealand to visit his brothers in Dunedin. He worked there and during this time became so engrossed with the theatre that he decided this was to be his career. He was in Melbourne for a short time, and in 1874 went to England with the sole purpose of becoming an actor. He obtained small parts, then for three and a half years was with Henry Irving, becoming his juvenile lead. After this, Bentley did some other stage work then became dissatisfied and decided he needed time for further study.

The following is a direct quote from Walter Bentley about this period of study, from an interview he gave for The Theatre Magazine, October 1st, 1915.
" ***Studies in the Highlands.***

I cancelled all my engagements. I went into the Highlands, to a shooting-box lent me by Bailie, of Douchflour, near Inverness, and there worked hard for six months. My study took the form of enquiry into the principles of elocution and the principles of gesture. I armed myself with all the recognised authorities - all the books dealing with elocution and gesture. Gradually I corrected my mistakes in these directions. I realised that the art of speech and the art of gesture should be co-ordinated - that one was of little use without the other; and that both arts should easily, naturally illustrate themselves in a man's acting. Briefly, the view I took - it is a view, by the way, that I have never since departed from - was that the more a man mastered the art of elocution and the art of gesture the more expressive, the more expositional must he be in his acting. ....

"Thus, elocution and gesture, properly employed, represent two factors that put the actor in the way of getting results which, without them, it would be impossible to achieve. .....

"Besides requiring the strengthening arts of elocution and gesture, the actor - that is, if he is to succeed in his profession - must be able to so shape or mould a character as to make it a telling creation with his audience".

Walter Bentley then returned to the stage, performing leading roles in Shakespeare and other plays, in England and America. In 1891 he returned to Australia to tour under the management of J. C. Williamson and George Coppin. His roles included Hamlet, David Garrick, Rob Roy and Matthias ('The Bells'.) The impact of Bentley's performances in Melbourne was strong and Table Talk, November 13th, 1891, noted: *"Since his sojourn in the Victorian capital Mr. Bentley has won great popularity. He has been made a member of the various leading clubs, and during the racing carnival he has been the guest of His Excellency Lord Hopetoun. Mr Bentley is an enthusiast at golf."*

Walter Bentley continued touring with great success for a number of years. Early in the 1900's he was back in England but from 1909 until his death in 1927 Walter Bentley lived in Sydney. There he taught elocution and dramatic art and was secretary, and president, for a time, of the Actors' Association of Australia. Ill-health dominated the last years of Walter Bentley's life, and he chose release from this by a bullet. A Sydney newspaper noted: *" Even in his private life Walter Bentley, known in the profession as "the Scotch Hamlet," carried an air of thespian tragedy. It was real tragedy that brought down the final curtain."*

Colleague

The name of R.F.Young was first associated with FM in Melbourne in 1900, when he was a tenant with FM on the seventh floor of the Australian Building, 49 Elizabeth Street. In 1901 the tenants of the fifth floor of the Equitable building in Sydney included FM Alexander and R.F.Young. The latter's advertisements included prominent reference to the " Sandow System of Physical Culture". R.F.Young's advertisements were often alongside those of FM.

That of February 16th, 1901 announced,

" **SANDOW'S SANDOW'S**

SYSTEM SYSTEM

of

HARMONIOUS PHYSICAL DEVELOPMENT
Mr. R. F. YOUNG'S
SCHOOL OF PHYSICAL CULTURE,

EQUITABLE BUILDING

"A SOUND MIND IN A SOUND BODY."

The Sandow System is recommended by LIEUT.-COLONEL FOX, Inspector of Gymnasia in Great Britain; SURGEON-MAJOR DEANS, Army Medical Staff.

Introduced into THE BRITISH ARMY, THE LONDON POLICE FORCE, THE LONDON FIRE BRIGADE ETC.

Mr. YOUNG having previously had many years' experience in all branches of Athletics, seven years' thorough gymnastic training, and possessing a knowledge of the anatomy of the human body, met Mr.Eugen Sandow in London in 1891, and after many interviews with him, and witnessing his work in private, was accorded the privilege of being present at a meeting of the medical profession when various tests were applied with astonishing results. Mr.Young, being convinced of its superiority, became an ardent STUDENT OF THE SANDOW SYSTEM, which he has already imparted to several members of the medical profession in Sydney.

The different modifications of the system enabled it to be applied to LADIES, CHILDREN, ATHLETES, THE DELICATE, and those who have reached the Meridian of Life.

The development is so symmetrical, the exercises so simple, and the danger of strain or fatigue so improbable that, with the aid of a teacher understanding, as Mr. Young does, the physiological law underlying all physical education, the average pupil at the end of a series is left in possession of sound lungs, a deep mobile chest, healthy organs, and an evenly balanced muscular and nervous system".

Eugen Sandow (1867 - 1935) was born in East Prussia. As a young man he developed the ability to perform prodigious feats of strength. His tours to exhibit his physical prowess led him in 1889 to England where he became a principle topic of conversation in sporting circles. Eugen Sandow established himself in England, where, as well as giving exhibitions as a strongman, and a showman, he opened various centres of Physical Culture to teach his methods. There were also numerous travels abroad, including Australia in 1902. Wherever Eugen Sandow went he gave lectures and demonstrations on Physical Culture to the various scientific, educational, medical, military, athletic and police authorities, as well as entertaining an admiring public with his feats of strength. His 1902 tour of Australia covered five states.

R.F.Young continued to advertise himself in Sydney as a teacher of the Sandow System. In the early part of 1904, FM Alexander went to England and R.F.Young remained at their shared studios to continue his Physical Culture school. On August 27th of that year R.F.Young advertised as follows:

" **SANDOW SYSTEM MR. R. F. YOUNG'S**
School of Physical Culture
Royal Chambers, Castlereagh Street

SPECIAL ANNOUNCEMENT

The leading members of the MEDICAL PROFESSION OF LONDON have expressed the opinion that

MR. F. MATTHIAS ALEXANDER'S SPECIAL BREATHING METHOD, as applied in the TREATMENT OF DISEASE *(under medical supervision),*

surpasses all methods at present known to them, and, in consequence, they have induced him to remain in London to receive the patients they are recommending for treatment.

The methods referred to are imparted by
Mr.YOUNG,

who has been associated with Mr.Alexander in his professional work for many years. The methods are imparted in their entirety by Mr.Young, who has successfully treated patients suffering with ASTHMATIC, THROAT, CHEST, HEART, NERVE, AND STOMACH Diseases, POST-NASAL (Adenoid) Growths, and the after-effects of PLEURISY etc.

Medical references. Write for Pamphlet".

On March 3rd 1906, an advertisement by R.F.Young for his Physical Culture School included the following: *" Alexander's Full-chest Breathing method, Pronounced by Leading Medical Men in London as surpassing all others in the treatment of disease, is imparted. London and Sydney Medical References."*

In 1908 R.F.Young had a business listing as follows:
" Young R.F. Sandow School of Physical Culture, Japanese Ju-Jitsu and Alexander's Breathing Method. Ladies, Gentlemen and Children. Angel Place, off 127 Pitt Street."

This listing remained until 1910.

In September of that year Robert F. Young died in Sydney. He was Melbourne born (1856). His parents were both from overseas; his father, Arthur Forbes Young, from Antwerp, Belgium, and his mother, Marie Antoinette Perrin, from Mauritius, Isle of France, had married in Hobart in 1855. Their son, Robert F. Young married Edith Mary Page (second eldest of a family of eight children) in Hobart in 1883. At that time he was a Civil Servant but he also pursued and developed various other skills. That of physical culture eventually became his main work in Sydney. After his death, his widow married FM in London in 1914.

Reference has already been made in this book (chapter 12, on Dr. Leeper) to physical culture and its place in schools. As FM shared teaching studios with R.F.Young in both Melbourne and Sydney he would have known details of Young's physical culture method and no doubt been familiar with other physical training methods of those times. FM went to England in June 1904, and it was not long before he was producing his own pamphlets detailing his ideas about the subject. In his four books varying degrees of space are given to the subject of physical culture.

The fourth book, The Universal Constant In Living (first printed in 1941), has a specific reference to FM's Australian years; *"In Australia over forty years ago, in the rooms of one of the best teachers of physical culture I have ever known, I had my first experience of observing the results of exercises designed to bring about "specific effects." Although I disagreed then, as I still do, with the principle underlying his and all such teaching, we were both impressed by the fact that the same set of exercises was responsible for quite different effects in different people. How could it be otherwise?"*

This reference to *"one of the best teachers of physical culture"* must have meant R. F. Young. He was the person with whom FM had had a long association, sharing performances (R. F. Young in his role as pianist), sharing teaching studios, and no doubt having many discussions about all aspects of physical culture, including breathing techniques and specific exercise methods.

A few years after his arrival in England FM printed three pamphlets relating to Physical Culture.

(1) Why "Deep Breathing" and Physical Culture Exercises do more Harm than Good (1908)
(2) Re-education of the Kinaesthetic Systems (Sensory Appreciation of Muscular Movement), Concerned with the Development of Robust Physical Well-Being (1908)
(3) Why We Breathe Incorrectly - Some points in connection with the Scientific Explanation of the Latest Developments in Breathing, Physical Culture, and Voice Production (1909)

In No. 1 FM states, *"To this end I will deal with four of the primary ideas or principles upon which teachers of physical culture and "deep breathing" obviously base their methods. They instruct the pupil -*

(a) "To assume a proper standing position, to be adopted in their exercises and in everyday life."
(b) "To draw in a `deep breath'."
(c) "To hold the breath for a certain time, say, while they count 5, 10 or 20."
(d) "To expel the air retained by forcing in some part of the chest or abdominal wall."

When enlarging on this FM details section (a) as follows: *"In the first place, to allow a pupil to assume, of himself, a certain standing position, means that his own perceptions and sensations are given the sole onus of bringing about the co-ordination upon which such standing position depends - an onus which they are quite unable to bear. The perceptions and sensations of all who need respiratory and physical re-education are, as I shall show later, absolutely unreliable. It is the teacher who should have the responsibility of certain detailed orders, the literal carrying out which will ensure for the pupil what is then the correct standing position for him. I emphasise this last, because no one stereotyped position can be correct for each and every pupil. When a person so employs the different parts of his body that one can speak of his "harmful position in standing or walking," it is only by causing the physical machinery to resume correct and harmonious working gradually, thus changing the position from time to time, that serious harm can be averted and satisfactory results secured. I may point out, moreover, than in trying to assume the "proper standing position" at the outset, the pupil unavoidably puts severe strain upon the throat, thereby paving the way for throat, ear, and eye disorders."*

No. 2 pamphlet, Re-education of the Kinaesthetic Systems, begins with the following:

" *EDUCATION*

" It is because the body is a machine that education is possible. Education is the formation of habits, a super-inducing of an artificial organisation upon the natural organisation of the body; so that acts, which at first require a conscious effort, eventually became unconscious and mechanical."

- HUXLEY

RE-EDUCATION

"It is because the body is a machine that (RE)education is possible. (RE)education is the formation of (NEW AND CORRECT) habits, a (RE-INSTATING of THE CORRECT) artificial organisation upon the natural organisation of the body; so that acts, which at first require conscious effort, eventually became unconscious and mechanical."

22, ARMY AND NAVY MANSIONS
109, VICTORIA STREET,
LONDON,
S.W."

Eight points are then itemised with further detail about some of them. The eight points are as follows:

1. "That when defects in the poise of the body, in the pose of the chest, in the use of the muscular mechanisms, and in the equilibrium are present in the human being the condition thus evidenced is an undue rigidity of parts of the muscular mechanisms associated with undue flaccidity of others. This undue rigidity is always found in those parts of the muscular mechanisms which are forced to perform duties other than those intended by nature, and are consequently ill-adapted for their function."

2. "That it is essential at the outset of re-education to bring about the relaxation of the unduly rigid parts of the muscular mechanisms in order to secure the correct use of the inadequately employed and wrongly co-ordinated parts."

3. *"That all conscious effort exerted in attempts at physical action causes, in the great majority of the people of today, such tension of the muscular system concerned as to lead to exaggeration rather than eradication of the defects already present."*

4. *"That a directly conscious effort in the performance of the exercises employed in the early stages of re-education (a) implies that the pupil relies upon his own faulty sensations (that is, he is realising his sensations) for guidance in the correct performance of such exercises - guidance which it is not in the power of the incoherent and often absolutely misleading sensations of the imperfectly co-ordinated subject to give; and (b) produces, as a result of the tension induced by such effort, thoracic rigidity and breathlessness - the one making the correct performance of the exercises impossible, the other interfering with the controlling forces concerned."*

5. *"That it is harmful for teacher and pupil alike if the latter is made to assume, during his exercises, what is usually considered the correct standing position. It is obvious that the same position cannot be correct for every human being, nor even for all who are properly co-ordinated."*

6. *"That in order to obviate the evils enunciated in the last two postulates the teacher must himself place the pupil in a position of mechanical advantage, from which the pupil, by the mere mental rehearsal of orders which the teacher will dictate, can insure the posture specifically correct for himself, although he is not, as yet, conscious of what that posture is."*

7. *"That the orders to be dictated by the teacher and mentally rehearsed by the pupil are of two kinds: —*

(a) Concerning definite inhibition.

(b) Concerning definite performance."

8. *"That in order to secure the results desired, it is essential to teach the pupil to rehearse the dictated orders, not to do exercises, i.e., to devote his attention to apprehending the instructions of his teacher — those means whereby he is to gain what he requires, and not, as he will be apt to do, to concentrate his thoughts upon the end sought. The orders are necessarily prior to their execution, and if those dictated by the teacher are correct for the particular case in hand, the mental realisation by the pupil will be automatically followed by their correct performance - a co-ordinated association with the ideo-motor impulses."*

No. 3 pamphlet refers to Dr. Alexander Leeper's Report on Physical Culture commissioned by the Teachers and Schools Registration Board of Victoria (printed 1909, see Chapter 12) and quotes an extract from it. The main thrust of this pamphlet is a detailed explanation by FM about the misconceptions of his work expressed by a London medical doctor and former pupil of his, Dr. Scanes Spicer.

FM, an Australian Abroad

In early 1904 FM again, via advertisement, reminded the public about his forthcoming book on Breathing, announcing that *"orders for subscription copies of his book, at 10s 6d will not be received after the end of this month. Those who wish to secure a copy after the end of February will be required to pay one güinea, the price at which the book will be published"*. The book was destined not to be published in Australia. For various reasons, FM decided the time was opportune for him to take his work to England. He had the encouragement of some prominent people, including leading doctors, and he left Australia in the first part of 1904.

Once in England FM was able to establish a successful teaching practice. Over the years he had had at various times, a small number of assistants who taught his work, some of whom continued to teach on their own. In 1931 FM started his first course to train others to teach his methods, there was an initial enrolment of seven people. Since then Alexander Technique teacher training schools have been established in several countries. FM Alexander's promised book of 1904 appeared in England in 1910 as 'Man's Supreme Inheritance'. It is worth noting that in this book and his later ones FM speaks critically of some aspects of the various modes of physical culture with which he was familiar. FM's three subsequent books were; 'Constructive Conscious Control of the Individual' (1923); 'The Use of the Self' (1932); and 'The Universal Constant in Living' (1941).

FM made lengthy teaching visits to America but England remained his home. Since his death in London in 1955 the work to which he devoted his life has continued to grow. The Alexander Technique is now taught in over thirty countries, including Australia. FM was keen that Australians should train with him in England, then return home. World War Two intervened, though one Australian, Alan Murray, was eventually able to study with FM and bring the Alexander Technique back to Australia in 1950: but F.Matthias Alexander never returned to the land of his birth.

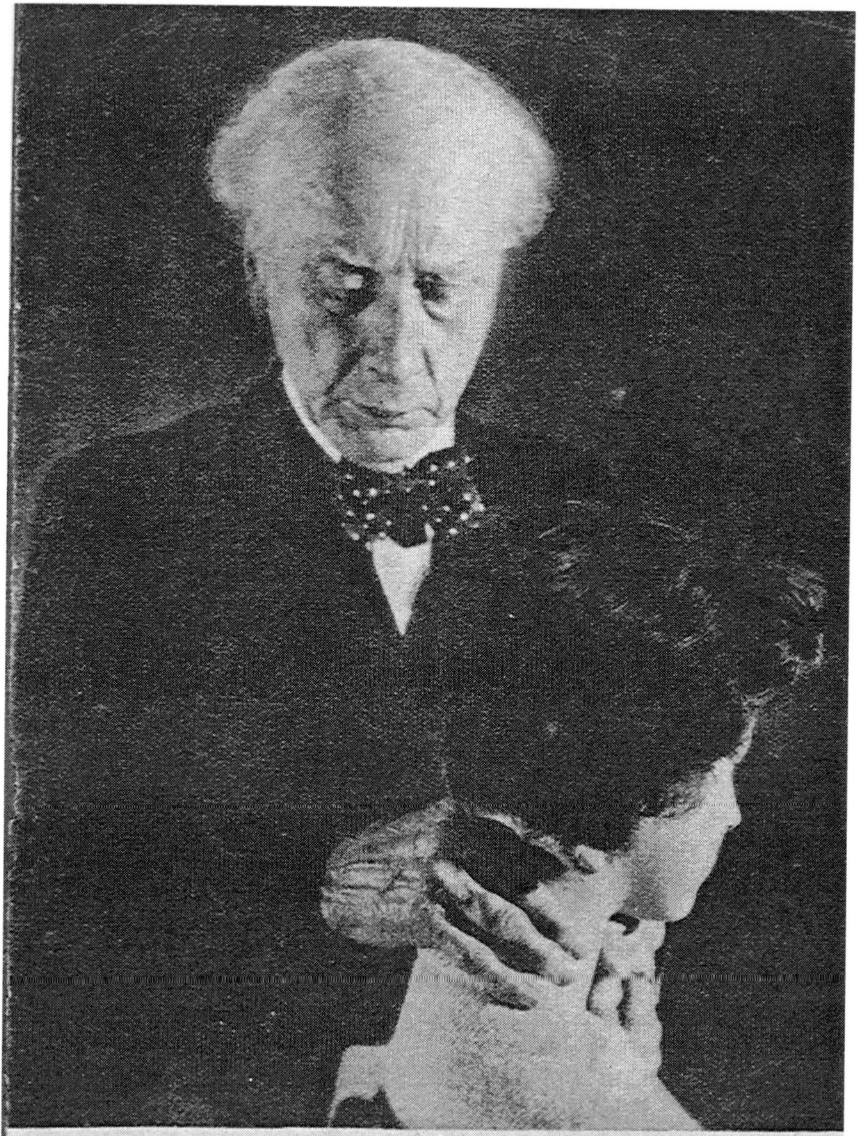

"Now to Stand Up"

The pupil must check her impulse to tense herself ready to get up.

The Master at Work (Leader Magazine, England, December 11th, 1948)

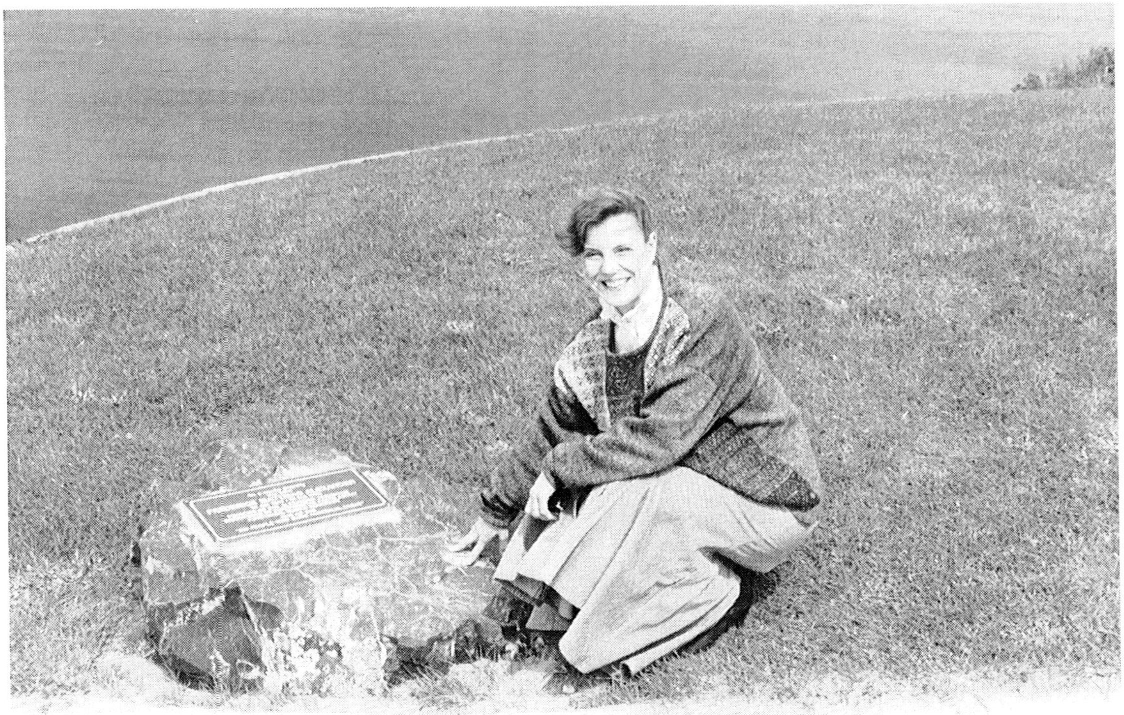

Plaque to FM Alexander on Table Cape Promontory, Tasmania
(Courtesy of Dr Ronald Wells and Janette Obuch Wells)

Appendix I

Poems FM recited

The Amateur Rider	*Banjo Paterson*
The Clock Mystery	*Rowe*
The Country Squire	*Anon.*
The Dream of Eugene Aram	*Thomas Hood*
In the Signal Box	*George R. Sims*
Keeping His Word	*Anon.*
Karl the Martyr	*Anon.*
Kissing Cup's Race	*Campbell Rae-Brown*
The Midnight Charge	*Clement Scott*
Parrhasius	*Nathaniel P. Willis*
Pat's Criticism	*Charles F. Adams*
The Progress of Madness	*Mathew G. Lewis*
Tim Twinkleton's Twins	*Anon.*
Wolf and Hound	*Charles A. Bell*
The Yarn of the "Nancy Bell"	*A. Lindsay Gordon*
	W. S. Gilbert

Appendix II

KISSING CUP'S RACE

You've never seen Kissing Cup—have you?
Stroll round to the paddock, my lord;
Just cast your eye over the mare, sir—
You'll say that, upon your word,
You ne'er saw a grander-shaped 'un
In all the whole course of your life.
Have you heard the strange story about her,
How she won Lord Hillhoxton his wife?

No? Well, if you've got a few minutes,
I'll tell you why Kissing Cup, here,
Has lived in this lazy grandeur
Since the first time they let her appear.
Here she is, sir; — now look her well over—
There isn't a fault to be found;
See her going— magnificent action !
You're right, sir; the mare is as sound
As she was on the day I rode her,
Just ten years ago last June:
I'll never forget how they cheered us,
The mare, and her jock, Bob Doon.

He was always a reckless youngster,
My master, Hillhoxton, you know;
And when the old Marquis died, sir,
He seemed—somehow or other—to go
Right fair clean away to the devil;
And, being a fresh 'un— you see? —
The "bookies" just fleeced him, a good'un—
I knew, sir, quite well how 'twould be;
I saw he would go down a mucker—
Be ruined, sir, sure as fate.
In his careless boyish folly

I saw that the fine old estate
Would be gambled away—the title
Be sullied, perchance, with shame.
I said to myself, "Bob Doon, boy,
You must save your old master's name."
He'd loved a quiet bit o'racing,
I'd been his head jock for years,
I remember the night he died sir:
His bright eyes filling with tears,
He told me to mind the youngster,
To see that he didn't begin
To gamble — and always remembered
The Hillhoxton's rode to win.
He told me, above all, to see, sir,
That no scandal e'er touched the stud;
To be sure that our stables harbour'd
Nought but the purest blood.
He took my rough hand as he finished
In the same old well known grip
As hundred of times I'd seen him
A-grasping the ribbons and whip.

He didn't last very much longer—
I stood by the bed as he died,
And watched my old master's spirit
Start on its last long ride

One night—I remeber it well sir—
It must have been just nigh four years
After the old Marquis left us—
Very heavy at heart with fears,
I was sitting in one of the stables,
Not dreaming as no one was near,
A-thinking of how things were looking
A mighty sight too deuced queer.
I had turned round my head for a moment
To see as the nags were all right,
When I saw the young master a-standing
Behind me. I started. The sight
Of his face, pale and haggard,
Sent a rush of cold blood to my heart.
I knew, sir, that something had happened.
"Doon, Doon, my boy, why do you start?

Don't you know me" he said. "Have I altered,
Have I changed! so since yesterday!
No wonder, good God! I am ruined!
I've gambled the old home away.
But the worst—the poor girl, Lady Constance—
You know how she loves me, old friend—
What will she think of me now, Bob?
For pity's sake, Heaven defend
And keep her," he cried, "true as ever!
But no, no! I can never wed
You now. God bless you, my darling!
Forget me as if I were dead."
He wept like a child in his sorrow.
"Be a man, be a man, sir," said I;
"Trust to me, I can yet pull you through, sir—
There's a mare in your stud that can fly.
I've kept her—I knew you were playing
Too fast, far too reckless, a game;
But there's Kissing Cup ready to run for
And save a Hillhoxton's name.

When I say that the lad was collected,
I asked him to turn and look
At the very first bet he had entered
On the very first page of his book.
He looked at me—eyes full of wonder—
"That's three years! What d'ye mean?"
"My lord, you'll forgive me," I answered;
"Forgive me, I know you have been
Too hot, aye, too heedless by far sir,
In your youthful and reckless career;
You've forgotten —just read for a moment
The words that you see written here."
I showed him the entry—five hundred
To one, clearly betted in "thous,"
Against the foal out of "Sweet Violet,"
By "Loving Cup," out of "Carouse."
The foal, Kissing Cup, here, is ready
And fit, sir, to run for a life;
In the big race next week she will save you,
Will win you a fortune — and wife."
The boy couldn't speak for a moment,
His pallid lips moved in a groan;

Then he rallied and grasping my hand, sir,
Held it just like a vice with his own.

The day of the race was a grand one,
But few knew the issue at stake;
We'd tried hard to keep it a secret
For the splendid old Marquis's sake,
As we cantered away past the stand, sir,
To give the "big swells" all a view,
Hardly one of 'em dreamt what 'twould mean sir,
If the Hillhoxton "Chocolate and Blue"
Were beaten—none guessed that the girl there,
With her beautiful face, worn and thin,
Was murmring a low prayer to Heaven
That her young lover's colours might win.

"All ready? — a beautiful start, sir;
The line was as straight as could be.
"They're off!" the shout rang for a moment
Around us, and then seemed to me
As dying away in the distance,
While we scudded along the course
At a pace that was far too killing
To last; so I kept my horse
Well back in the rear to "the Corner."
Then I let the reins loose on her mane.
She passed through them all but just one, sir,
Lort Rattlington's colt, Sugar Cane.
Then I saw there would be a struggle:
I had known it for months long back,
That all as I need be afraid of
Was the old Baron's fast-flying "crack."
'Twas a terrible moment for me, sir;
The colt was three good lengths ahead.
I whispered a word to the mare, sir:
'Twas enough—she knew what I said.
Sweeping on down the hill like a rocket,
She got to the girths of the colt.
My heart gave a great throb of pleasure,
"I made sure that he'd "shot his bolt."
But no! his jock hustled him up sir;
His whip swishes fell like rain,

And the cry ran like fire up the course, sir,
"It's thousands on Sugar Cane."
The stand was reached, Sugar Cane leading;
Two seconds and all would be o'er.
"Lord Rattlington wins!" No, not yet, though;
We're neck, sir to neck—two strides more.
I saw in the great sea of faces
A girl's—pale, white as the dead—
I cried, "For God's sake, Kissing Cup, now!"—

'Twas over—we'd won by a head!

Campbell Rae-Brown

Kissing Cup's Race was one of FM's favourite poems. It was written by Campbell Rae-Brown in England in the later part of the nineteenth century. This poem became very popular, not only as a piece for recitals, but also with those who loved romantic ballads.

ACKNOWLEDGMENTS

F.M.Alexander said that people generally were end-gainers, meaning that they were too intent on the goal and that not enough attention was paid to the means-whereby the goal was being achieved. Having goals is important but it is true that we must also look after ourselves during a time of endeavour and as much as possible keep in mind what we do with ourselves as we work towards a given goal.

The idea for a book about the Australian origins of FM has been in my mind for some years. Over time I have collected bits of information, it seemed appropriate with the growing interest in the historical aspects of the Alexander Technique to release in book form the information I have gathered. During the book's preparation I have no doubt, when working to deadlines, that at times I have been caught up in end-gaining and not paying enough attention to the means-whereby. However, thought is quick, remembrance of Alexander's principles is simple to return to, and reapplying them provides access to this most useful knowledge about the Use of the Self.

For the creation of this book I am indebted to the following organisations and individuals.The Archives of: Australian Medical Association, the Baptist Union of Victoria; the Uniting Church in Australia; Melbourne Girls Grammar; Presbyterian Ladies College; Registered Schools Board; Scotch College; Trinity College, Melbourne University; the Baillieu Library, Melbourne University; the State Library of Tasmania. Finally for two places where I spent many fascinating and at times fruitful hours of research: the Public Records Office in Melbourne and the State Library of Victoria, especially the La Trobe Reference Centre.

There are many individuals who have given encouragement and support, I am grateful to all those people. They include: Helen Clark, Alicia Gleeson, Anna Gleeson, Peter Keenan, Kiera Lindsey, Pam Lockhart, Cindy Louey, Denise Mancini, Jim Alexander, Ken Alexander, Mrs Butler, Dr.Ruth Campbell, Mrs Dutton, Anne Edgeworth, Margaret Long, Janette Obuch, Marion Poynter and Dr.Ailsa Zainu'ddin.

The following list of articles and pamphlets by F.M.Alexander have been quoted by kind permission of © The Estate of F.M.Alexander 1995.

"Elocution as an Accomplishment" (1894) Page 59
"Speech Culture and Natural Elocution" (1895) Page 62

"Why Deep Breathing and Physical Culture Exercises do more Harm than Good" (1908) Page 134

"Re-education of the Kinaesthetic Systems (Sensory Appreciation of Muscular Movement), Concerned with the Development of Robust Physical Well-Being" (1908) Page 134

"Why We Breathe Incorrectly - Some points in connection with the Scientific Explanation of the Latest Developments in Breathing, Physical Culture, and Voice Production." (1909) Page 134

The idea for a book and its fulfilment needs not only planning and writing but also the all important aspect of editing and preparation from the manuscript to the type-set page. Jocelyn Terry has most obligingly been critic and encourager in her role as Editor. Alex Kaplan has willingly assisted in preparation of the manuscript for printing, and with research, her help made it possible for me to meet the necessary publishing deadline. I am especially grateful to these two people whose support enabled my dream to become a reality.

BIBLIOGRAPHY

Concise History of Australia — Russel Ward

Australia, the Creation of a Nation. — Charles Wilson

Captain Swing — E. J. Hobsbawm & George Rude

Bush Life in Tasmania — James Fenton

And Wealth for Toil — Kerry Pink

Marvellous Melbourne — Graeme Davison

James Smith,the making of a Colonial Culture — Lurline Stuart

Entertaining Australia, the Performing Arts as Cultural History — Ed. Katherine Brisbane

Theatre in Australia — John West

Every Little Movement — Ted Shawn

The four books by F.M.Alexander are:

Man's Supreme Inheritance
Constructive Conscious Control of the Individual
The Use of the Self
Universal Constant in Living

Of the more than twenty books about the Alexander Technique, one of the best is, Body Awareness in Action by Frank Pierce-Jones.

Books about the Alexander Technique are certainly worth reading but are best used initially as an adjunct to practical Alexander study. Alexander teachers now work in over thirty countries. Phone books usually have listings under **Alexander Technique**, as to contact points for Alexander Societies and individual teachers.